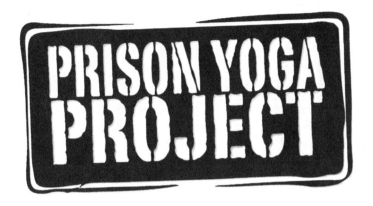

A PATH FOR HEALING
AND RECOVERY

JAMES FOX

The Prison Yoga Project wishes to thank the Give Back Yoga Foundation (www.givebackyoga.org) for their dedicated financial support of the printing and distribution of this book.

Any sales or donations related to the book go toward supporting the Prison Yoga Project's efforts to establish yoga and meditation practices in prisons and rehabilitation facilities.

Artwork: cover, pages 5, 23 and 84/85. Brett Crawford
Illustrations: pages 12, 14, 16, 18, 20 and 21;
24, 26, 28, 30, 32, 34 and 35; 38, 40, 42, 44, 46, 48 and 49; 54, 56, 58, 60, 62, 64, 66, 68, 70, 72 and 73. Ben Ballard
Graphic Design: Geoliphic Media

ISBN: 978-1-61623-839-1

Prison Yoga Project
P.O. Box 415
Bolinas, CA 94924
http://prisonyoga.org

Introduction

This book is inspired by the Prison Yoga Project's mission to support the practice of yoga and mindful awareness in prisons and rehabilitation facilities worldwide. This is the second edition of the book with added information and asana practices. It is published in response to thousands of inquiries from prisoners everywhere for a guide to yoga, as well as to provide my students at California's San Quentin Prison with a yoga practice they can continue upon their release.

These practices have proven effective in helping prisoners to gain insight into unconscious patterns of thinking and compulsive behavior. They have also greatly helped in improving their overall quality of life - mentally, emotionally and physically. Although this program has been developed through years of experience teaching yoga to incarcerated youth and adults, it focuses on the self-reflection and personal discipline necessary for one to lead a more conscious life, whether incarcerated or free. It is a powerful resource for anyone trying to break free of negative behavioral patterns.

The practices in this booklet develop and nurture one's "inner guide" or "true self" that has the ability and strength to witness and respond with awareness to situations and circumstances that arise, rather than reacting blindly to them. Although the ultimate purpose of these practices is to expand one's consciousness and increase life force energy, they also serve as a practical tool for developing impulse control, particularly as it relates to managing emotions and curbing addictive tendencies.

Yoga offers an alternative way of being with yourself and the world. It represents a personal support system that if practiced regularly can provide you with an ongoing sense of balance, connectedness and inner peace. To heal the pain and suffering in the world requires us to heal our own pain and suffering, so we no longer unconsciously inflict pain and suffering on others. May this book assist you on your path of self-discovery, healing and true liberation.

James Fox
Bolinas, California

Why Yoga in Prison?

"The memory of trauma is imprinted on the human organism. I don't think you can overcome it unless you learn to have a friendly relationship with your body." Bessel van der Kolk, M.D., Professor of Psychiatry, *Boston University School of Medicine, and pioneer researcher in the field of trauma.*

Prison is a breeding ground for mental, emotional and physical distress. Experiences of anxiety, depression, fear, distrust, agitation, hopelessness, grief, and violence can be greatly increased under incarcerated conditions. Psychiatrists, psychologists and clinical social workers acknowledge that embodiment practices such as yoga can greatly help people alleviate the symptoms that lead to both reactive behaviors and stress-related disease. So learning a practice in prison for Mindful Awareness and embodiment is not only important for supporting behavioral rehabilitation, it is also critical for physical and emotional well being.

Dr. Van der Kolk's quote above illustrates that to heal from the emotional and sometimes physical pain of trauma requires establishing a meaningful connection with our hearts and bodies. Most people in prison have become dissociated from their feelings and bodies as a result of backgrounds of trauma including neglect or abuse, violent behavior, and/or the overuse of drugs and alcohol. The convict code can further distance one from a meaningful connection with his body, emotions and deeper self. Yoga helps to become more sensitive to yourself because it is a practice of self-awareness and self-control that promotes non-reactivity and self-acceptance. A regular yoga practice can help free the mind from confusion and the body from distress, allowing one to be at peace and receptive to learning new ways of thinking, feeling and being. Yoga emphasizes discipline of the mind and body for developing positive behavioral habits and impulse control.

The most often reported benefits from students involved in Prison Yoga Project classes are:

- Reduction of stress
- "More able to focus on the positive rather than the negative"
- Support in addiction recovery
- Greater mental clarity
- Pain relief
- Improved sleep
- "Better able to deal with the mental and emotional strain of prison"
- Greater access to inner peace

Origins of Yoga

The word "yoga" is derived from the Sanskrit word meaning to bind or join. In philosophical terms this refers to the union of the body with the mind, as well as the mind with a pure state of consciousness. Contrary to popular belief, yoga practices are not tied specifically to Hindu theology or Buddhist philosophy. Although written about in many of the ancient Hindu scriptures including the Vedas and the Bhagavad Gita, the common ancestors of yoga were ascetics and shamans who used various physical and psychological exercises as vehicles to realize heightened states of consciousness.

Yoga involves disciplined introspection with the aim of freeing oneself from identification with the ego. There are many forms of yoga including: *bhakti* yoga, the yoga of devotion; *jnana* yoga, the yoga of knowledge; *karma* yoga, the yoga of action; and *raja* yoga, the yoga of psychological/physical exercise.

Raja Yoga

The type of yoga presented in this book is *raja* ("royal") yoga, which is based upon some of the earliest writings on the practice of yoga found in an ancient text called the Yoga Sutra, believed to have been written sometime around 250 B.C by a wise man named Patanjali. The methodology for *raja* yoga, also known as classical yoga, follows an eight-fold path outlined in the Yoga Sutra called the Eight Limbs that offer step-by-step instructions about how a person can find inner peace and knowledge through yoga (*see Eight Limbs, pages 7 & 8*). Patanjali did not attribute his instructions to any particular religion or philosophy but rather advocated the practice of yoga for living a moral, self-disciplined and meaningful life.

Raja yoga involves disciplining the mind, body and emotions to disengage from identification with the ego (the personal self), and achieve a state of higher consciousness for the specific purpose of self-realization, i.e. realizing one's true nature or Self. It includes the practice of postures (*asanas*), conscious breathing (*pranayama*) and meditation (*dhyana*).

One of the original purposes for practicing raja yoga was to prepare the mind and body for periods of prayer or meditation. Another was to develop the mental, emotional and physical discipline as well as spiritual values required of traditional warriors. In most tribal communities, warriors have always been those the community could count on for protection, and unlike today, their focus was on developing defensive skills rather than offensive ones, using force only as a last resort.

While there are currently many approaches to the practice of yoga, most embody a sophisticated system of exercises and stretches, or postures (*asanas*) combined with conscious breathing (*pranayama*) that can create a strong sense of physical, mental and emotional well being. The practice improves physical balance, flexibility and stamina while mentally and emotionally generating self-awareness and a sense of calmness. Unlike other forms of exercise that can strain muscles and bones, the intention of yoga is to rejuvenate the body and free the mind from tension brought about by the stress of life.

Mindful Awareness

Mindful awareness (also known as mindfulness) is at the very core of a yoga practice. Mindful awareness involves using the mind for a different purpose than thinking thoughts. Rather it focuses the mind on feeling sensations in the body and the movement of the breath. It is a practice of keeping the mind steady by paying close attention to what's going on moment-to-moment. It involves being present in each moment allowing the mind to observe rather than interpret what is going on. Mindful awareness can be practiced in seated meditation and while actively engaged in *asana* practice. The main components that constitute mindful awareness are:

- Learning to relax into a state of awareness and connecting with sensations in the body.
- Releasing involvement with thoughts and instead focusing on the movement of the breath while breathing through the nose.
- Practicing simply observing or witnessing one's moment-to-moment experience.

Thanks to research at the University of Massachusetts Medical Center, UCLA's Mindful Awareness Research Center, Harvard University and other prestigious institutes, mindful awareness has scientific support as a means for reducing stress, improving attention, boosting the immune system and promoting a general sense of psychological and physical well-being. Case studies have also shown that mindful awareness is effective in increasing self-esteem and holds great promise for both adolescents and adults with ADHD, depression, anxiety and other mood disorders.

Postures (*Asanas*)

The postures or *asanas* that are employed in the practice of *raja* yoga are what most people in America think of as yoga. However in actuality they only represent one of the Eight Limbs. The stretches, twists, bends, inversions and other postures that comprise the *asana* practice, along with conscious breathing (*pranayama*), are intended to cleanse and purify all the systems of the body removing obstructions to the flow of life force energy. While appearing to deal with the physical body alone, *asanas* and *pranayama* actually influence the nervous system and the chemical balance of the brain. So practicing yoga not only restores strength and stamina to the body but also can help improve one's mental and emotional states.

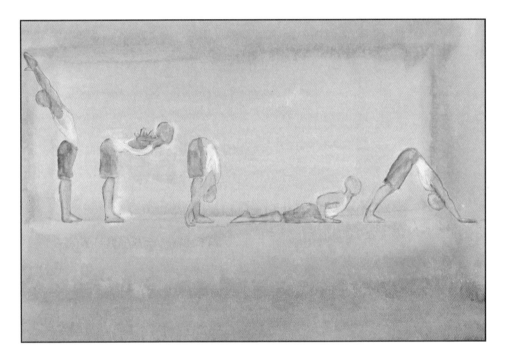

Probably the most well recognized series of asanas is Surya Namaskara, or Sun Salutations. These could be commonly described as "yoga calisthenics," and variations of these are included as a part of almost any yoga practice.

Conscious Breathing (Pranayama)

Pranayama, the practice of conscious control of breathing, is another main component of *Raja* Yoga. *Prana* is the yogic word for the life force energy that permeates the individual, all living beings and life forms, as well as the air we breathe. *Ayama* is the storing or movement of that energy. So *pranayama* is the practice of influencing the flow of life force energy in and through the body using the breath.

Our main source of *prana* comes from the air we breathe, and the amount of *prana* we circulate through our bodies greatly impacts our overall vitality. The very basics of *pranayama* involve focused awareness on both inhale and exhale, breathing through the nose, and relaxing and stabilizing the breath to support the asana practice. Exhalation becomes consciously connected to letting go or releasing. Depending on the specific practice, engaging in *pranayama* can increase energy or provide calmness and clarity.

See the Pranyama section in this book (pgs. 76-83) for more details about specific practices.

THE EIGHT LIMBS OF YOGA
A PATH FOR THE COMMITTED PRACTITIONER

The main goal of yoga is to free the mind from confusion and distress allowing oneself to be at peace, and from that state sink into deeper levels of awareness to experience one's true nature or Being. As discussed previously, there are eight (*ashto*) fundamental principles of *raja* yoga known as limbs (*anga*) that serve as a path for the committed practitioner.

1. *Yama* - meaning "restraint," explains the codes of ethical behavior to be observed in everyday life reminding us of our personal responsibilities. They involve how we interact with people and the environment. *Yama*, consists of five principles:
- *Ahimsa* or non-violence that requires introspection to replace negative, destructive thoughts and actions with positive constructive ones. *Ahimsa* is more than a lack of violence. It includes kindness, friendliness and thoughtful consideration. And importantly, *Ahimsa* also includes kindness toward ourselves.
- *Asteya* or freedom from avarice; not stealing or taking what is not offered.
- *Satya* means to speak the truth. However in considering this, if speaking the truth has negative consequences for another, then it is better to say nothing.
- *Brahamacharya* or chastity, not total abstinence but rather a disciplined sexual life promoting contentment and moral strength within.
- *Aparigraha* or freedom from greed and possessiveness; that we take only what is necessary.

2. *Niyama* – compared to the *Yamas*, *Niyamas* are more intimate and personal. They refer to the attitude we adopt toward ourselves. *Niyamas* involve the positive current that brings discipline, removes inertia and gives shape to the inner desire to follow a yogic path. The principles of *Niyama* are:
- *Saucha* or cleanliness.
- *Santosa* means contentment, or more importantly to accept what happens.
- *Tapas* literally means to heat the body and by so doing to cleanse it. *Tapas* involve self-discipline with the desire to purify the body, senses and mind.
- *Svadhyaya* means self-inquiry, self-reflection, studying oneself to include the body, mind, intellect and ego.
- *Isvarapranidhana* literally means surrendering to the God of your understanding; offering the fruits of one's daily actions in service to a higher power.

3. *Asana* – are postures intended to generate, organize and distribute energy while focusing the attention inward to sharpen control of the mind and body. These series of exercises are intended to purify both physical and mental faculties and remove energetic blockages. A turning point in the practice of *asanas* is when one experiences the body, mind and spirit (or inner Self) united.

4. *Pranayama* – is control of inner life force energy by use of conscious breathing. It involves the expansion of this vital force energy, and is interrelated and interwoven with *asanas*. *Pranayama* has three basic movements: deep inhalation, complete exhalation, and full awareness of the pauses in between the two.

5. *Pratyahara* – evolves from *pranayama* and *asana* practice and represents detachment from or restraint of the senses, as the mind turns inward.

6. *Dharana* – is concentration of the mind's attention on a single thought or a "spot."

7. *Dhyana* – means "meditation; contemplation." It is a prolonged concentration of the mind as it remains focused and expanded into quietness. *Dhyana* frees an individual from attachment to the joys of pleasure or the sorrows of pain.

8. *Samadhi* – is a state of total absorption experienced at the level of the heart when oneness becomes realized (superconsciousness or Self-realization). The meditation and the meditator become one and awareness of an individual self is lost resulting in freedom from matter and thought.

Yamas and *niyamas* are the basic ethical trainings required of a committed yoga practitioner. As these become established an individual will begin to realize the fruits of his practice; without these it will not bear fruit. A yogi does not think of injuring anyone by thought, word or action.

Asana and *pranayama* represent the physical limbs of yoga. They are practiced to awaken the vital force energy of the body (*prana* or *chi*) and stimulate the nerve currents to travel up the spine, the *sushumna*, to illuminate the brain and impact one's "state of mind." *Asana* and *pranayama* are to be practiced regularly to purify and cleanse both the mind and the body, and provide for an expansion of consciousness that facilitates experiencing *pratyahara, dharana, dhyana and samadhi. Dharana, dhyana* and *samadhi* all involve the integration of the body, breath, mind, and Self.

These eight limbs represent a path for an individual's journey toward Self-realization and true freedom - freedom from matter and thought. Each limb is to be contemplated and practiced with patience, discipline and self-acceptance to experience the ultimate goal of yoga, freedom from the prison of the mind and realization of one's true being or Self.

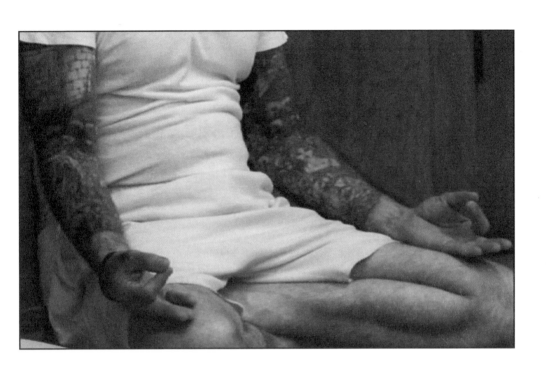

Preparation for Practice

In preparation to perform the yoga sessions presented in this booklet, it is best that you avoid eating a full meal up to three hours before practicing. If necessary, you can have a light snack no less than an hour before beginning. Do not drink water or other liquids during your practice. On the days you do your *asana* practice try to remember to drink plenty of water afterwards to facilitate detoxification and the cleansing process. Wear loose, comfortable clothing for ease of movement. It is ideal to practice barefoot on a clean floor using a yoga mat, though a blanket could be substituted for a mat. Given the opportunity, it is also wonderful to practice outside on grass or a soft surface.

It is extremely important to breathe through your nose when practicing yoga unless you are unable to do so because of injury or illness. Breathing through the nose allows the hairs in the nostrils to filter out particles of dust and dirt that can be harmful to the lungs. If too many particles become trapped on the membranes of the nose, the body secretes mucus to expel them. Also, the mucous membranes of the septum that separate the two nostrils serve to warm the air for our lungs.

Another important reason to breathe through the nose is to maintain the proper balance of oxygen and carbon dioxide in our blood. When breathing through the mouth, we normally inhale and exhale air quickly and in large volumes. Research has shown that releasing carbon dioxide too quickly can cause arteries and blood vessels to constrict, not allowing the oxygen in our blood to reach the cells in sufficient quantity. Lack of sufficient oxygen going to the cells of the brain can trigger the sympathetic nervous system that accelerates the heart and triggers a "fight or flight" response, making us feel tense and irritable. When breathing through the nose we are more apt to inflate the entire lung and engage the parasympathetic nervous system that slows the heart rate, relaxes and calms the body. The sympathetic and parasympathetic nervous systems comprise the two divisions of the autonomic nervous system, which is the motor division of our general nervous system that regulates organs and other functions such as heart rate, digestion and breathing without conscious effort.

Introduction to Practices

There are several, complete yoga *asana* practices illustrated throughout the following pages, ranging from beginning to somewhat advanced. These are offered based on their effectiveness in prison classes with a variety of students with different physical and psychological issues. Ideally they should be practiced regularly at least three to four times a week. The order or sequencing of the *asanas* compliments the effects of each pose while maximizing the benefits of the practice. Each routine should take between 60-90 minutes and can generally be divided into six areas of focus:

Centering – the initial 5 to 10 minutes is devoted to establishing the foundation of mindful awareness for the practice by disengaging from preoccupations of the mind and initiating the conscious breath work that is integral for the practice.

Opening - the experience of centering is enhanced by engaging in a series of preliminary poses intended to begin stimulating the flow of life-force energy (*prana*) through the entire body while maintaining focused awareness on the breath.

Purification - this segment of the practice is intended to purify the mind and body through a vigorous set of rhythmic postures that involve repetitive movement and muscular contraction. Continued concentrated breathing is important to support the body through this energetic cleansing process.

Resiliency - this period involves building core physical, mental and emotional fortitude through a set of predominantly standing poses that develop balance and stamina.

Closing - this part of the practice is dedicated to penetrating deeply into the mind and body, holding postures for longer periods of time to stimulate the flow of energy to the joints, connective tissue and organs, calming the nervous system and preparing to move into stillness.

Integration - this final segment is devoted to surrendering the mind and body to stillness, integrating the physical, mental and emotional benefits of the practice.

Throughout your session it is important to practice mindful awareness as much as possible. This requires focusing awareness on and feeling the movement of the breath and sensations in the body rather than evaluating what is happening. If or when you find while you are practicing that your awareness has drifted off into thinking, planning, critiquing, judging, etc. - bring yourself back to the sensations in your body and your breathing. Feel deeply into yourself as you perform the poses, keeping your awareness on your breath to anchor yourself into the moment.

Simple Practice

The Simple Practice is for those who may have physical issues limiting them from practicing a more active or vigorous style of yoga. Nonetheless it provides a variety of fundamental asanas intended to introduce the practitioner to the intention and benefits of yoga. The Simple Practice as illustrated and described should take between 45-60 minutes to complete.

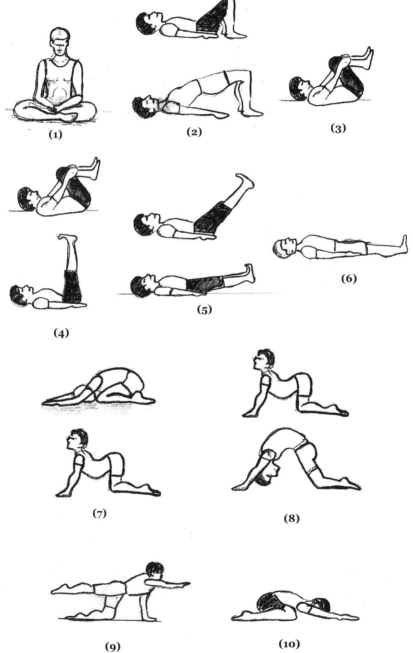

(1)

(2)

(3)

(4)

(5)

(6)

(7)

(8)

(9)

(10)

Centering & Opening

(1) Easy Pose (*Sukhasana*) - seated in cross-legged position allow the spine to lengthen gently toward the crown of the head; chest open, shoulders relaxed. Chin dropped slightly toward the chest, head positioned so openings of ears are aligned with the shoulder joints. Shift weight slightly forward on sitting bones to stabilize arch in the lower back. Proper alignment assists in keeping the body stable and still, supporting meditation practice. If unable to sit in this position, you can sit on a chair with your back supported. *Sit quietly for 5 minutes (see Daily Meditation Practice or Expanding Awareness of Breath).*

(2) Bridge (*Setu Banda Sarvangasana*) - come lying down on your back. Extend your arms along side your body. Bend your legs and walk your feet in close to your buttocks. Keeping your feet and knees hip width apart. Inhale and lift the hips and buttocks pressing the soles of your feet into the floor. As you exhale, slowly roll the spine down one vertebra at a time. Continue moving with your breath, rising on inhale, lowering on exhale. After 5-6 repetitions, rise up into the bridge, walk your shoulder blades in toward one another, press your arms against the floor and stay in the pose. Keep pressing the feet into the floor engaging the muscles of the legs, buttocks and back to keep the body lifted. *Stay at least 5 complete breaths before rolling back down on your back.*

NOTE: poses 3-6 are done as a continuous set.

(3) Knees to Chest (*Apanasana*) - staying on your back lift your feet off the floor. With your arms extended, hold onto your knees (shoulder width apart) or upper shins. Inhale fully and as you exhale completely out your nose, draw your knees into your chest. *Repeat at least 3-4 times.*

(4) Legs 90° to Floor - after exhaling and drawing your knees toward your chest, inhale and raise your legs perpendicular (90°) to the floor, feet together. Keep your quadriceps muscles and feet flexed, toes curling toward your shins as you extend the heels toward the ceiling. Exhale completely as you draw your knees in toward your chest. *Repeat 3-4 times.*

(5) Abdominal/Core Strength Building - from your legs raised 90° to the floor with feet together, lower the legs halfway to the floor (from 90o to 45°). Keep your legs and feet flexed as you extend out through your heels. *Try holding to the count of 10 before lowering the heels to the floor.*

(6) Resting - separate your feet hip width apart; rest your hands on your lower belly below the navel. Let your legs and feet roll open. Pick you head up and lengthen your neck tucking your chin toward your chest before resting the back of the head on the mat. Feel your belly rising and falling under your hands with each breath, let yourself relax completely, keeping your awareness on your breathing rather than thoughts.

NOTE: Poses 7-8 are done as a continuous set.

(7) Child's Pose (*Balasana*) to Cow - spread knees hip width apart and sit back toward your heels with your arms out in front of you. Keep the spine lengthened as you rest your forehead on the mat. Inhale and slowly begin to rise onto your hands and knees letting your head be the last part of the body that comes up into Cow pose. Allow your back and spine to arch, tale bone tilted upward, belly relaxed, arms straight with wrists under shoulders and knees under hips. Tilt head back looking up toward eyebrows. As you exhale, slowly come back to Child's Pose, letting your head be the last part of your body that comes down as you look toward the tip of your nose. Continue moving back and forth from Child's Pose to Cow (*4-5 repetitions*), always moving with inhale and exhale as described.

(8) Cow/Cat - from Cow, rather than going back to Child's pose, as you exhale transition to Cat, rounding the spine and back, drawing the lower belly in toward the spine, tucking the tailbone between the legs, bringing your chin to the collarbone, looking to the tip of your nose. As your chin comes to your collarbone complete the exhale expelling all the air from the lungs. *4-5 repetitions.*

(9) Sunbird (*Chakravakasana*) – starting with wrists under shoulders and knees under hips, hip width apart, reach your right arm straight out in front of you, and lift and extend your left leg straight back behind you. Right arm and left leg parallel to floor extending out through fingertips and toes. Then switch reaching forward with left arm and lifting the right leg. *Duration: 5 complete breaths each side, breathing slowly through the nose.*

(10) Child's Pose - spread knees wide apart, drop buttocks toward floor. Keep the spine lengthened as you rest your forehead on the mat or a rolled up towel. Arms can be resting out in front of you or alongside your legs. *Duration: at least 10 complete, deep, relaxing breaths.*

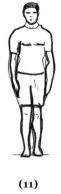

(11)

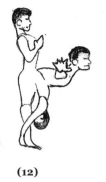

(12)

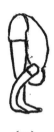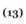

(13)

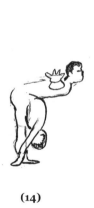

(14)

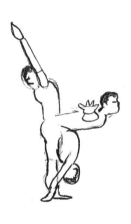

(15)

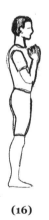

(16)

Opening (continued)

(11) Mountain (*Tadasana*) - keeping your legs flexed, weight balanced on your feet, hip width apart, spine lengthened, shoulder blades slightly together and arms dangling along your side, close your eyes. Staying grounded through the soles of your feet, focus all of your awareness on the sensation of your breath moving in and out of the nose. *Duration: 5-10 complete breaths.*

(12) Mountain to Standing Forward Fold – bring your hands together in front of your heart at your sternum. Pause for a breath or two. Then upon inhaling, sweep your arms out to the side raising them so that your hands come together over your head. Look to your hands, and upon exhaling, fold forward keeping the spine lengthened while sweeping the arms downward along side your body and settling into the forward fold.

(13) Standing Forward Fold (*Uttanasana*) – remaining in Standing Forward Fold, you can bend your knees slightly keeping the legs and feet hip width apart. Keep your weight evenly balanced on your feet from side to side and heel to toes. Try flexing your legs as you allow the torso to fold over the legs, spine lengthening toward the crown of your head. *Duration: 5 complete breaths.*

(14) Standing Half Forward Fold (*Ardha Uttanasana*) - from Standing Forward Fold, on an inhale bring your back up parallel with the floor first extending your arms out to the side; arms, back of head and neck and spine all in parallel alignment. *Duration: 3 complete breaths.*

(15 & 16) Transition to Standing - from Standing Half Forward Fold, inhale and raise the torso keeping the spine lengthened, sweeping the arms up from the sides of the body until the palms of the hands meet over head. Look to your hands above your head, and as you exhale extend the arms out to the side and down. Then bring your palms together to your sternum (heart) in a prayer gesture. *Stay here for 5 complete breaths.*

NOTE: *repeat poses 12-16 twice more.*

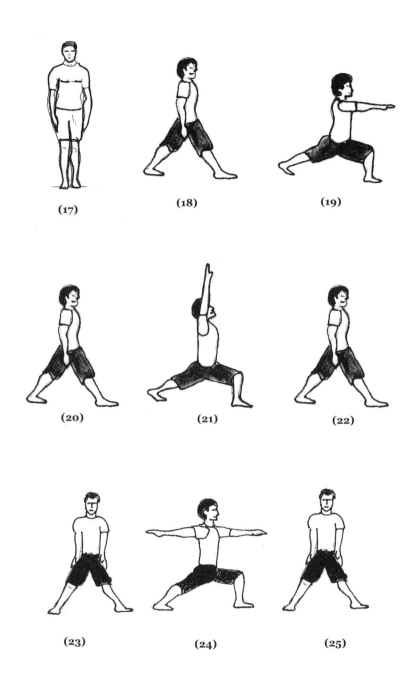

(17)   (18)   (19)

(20)   (21)   (22)

(23)   (24)   (25)

Resiliency

NOTE: poses 18-22 are done as a continuous set.

(17) Mountain (*Tadasana*) - keeping your legs flexed, weight balanced on your feet, hip width apart, spine lengthened, shoulder blades slightly together and arms dangling along your side, close your eyes. Staying grounded through the soles of your feet, focus all of your awareness on the sensation of your breath moving in and out of the nose *Duration: 5 complete breaths.*

(18, 19 & 20) Warrior I Prep - from Mountain Pose step the right foot back 3-4 feet, keeping it angled forward. Try to maintain heel-to-heel alignment of the feet, from front to back. Hips should be squared, facing forward. Inhale and bend the left leg as close to 90° as possible while raising the arms chest high in front of you. Exhale and straighten the left leg while bringing your arms alongside your body. *Repeat 4 times moving with the breath as described.* The fourth time hold pose 19 for three breaths before exhaling while bringing your arms alongside your body.

(21 & 22) Warrior I (*Virabhadrasana I*) - from pose 20 (see description above), when next inhaling, bend the left leg and raise your arms overhead keeping the right leg straight and right foot firmly planted on the mat. Exhale and straighten the left leg while bringing your arms alongside your body (pose 22). *Repeat 4 times, moving with the breath as described.* The fourth time hold pose 21 (Warrior I) for three breaths before exhaling while bringing your arms alongside your body.

NOTE: Repeat poses 18-22 as described but with left foot back and right foot forward.

(23, 24 & 25) Warrior II (*Virabhadrasana II*) - from pose 22, turn your right foot to the side, and open your hips in the same direction. Feet should be 4-5 ft. apart. Your front heel should be aligned with the middle of the arch of the back foot, the back foot angled slightly forward. Inhale and bring your arms up parallel with the floor as you bend the left leg as close to a 90° angle as possible. Your left knee should be directly over your left ankle. Keep the back leg straight lengthening it and pressing the back foot firmly into the mat. Look to the tips of your left fingers. Keep your torso vertically aligned over your hips. Exhale and straighten the left leg, bringing your arms alongside your body resting hands on thighs. *Repeat 4 times, moving with the breath as described.* The fourth time, stay in pose 24 (Warrior II) for three full breaths before exhaling while bringing your arms alongside your body.

NOTE: Repeat poses 23-25 as described but with left leg back and right leg forward. Look to right fingertips in pose 24.

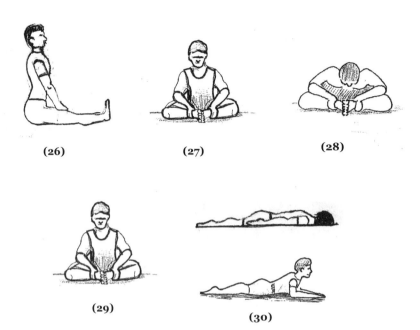

(26)   (27)   (28)

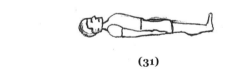

(29)   (30)

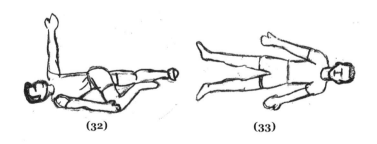

(31)

(32)   (33)

18

Closing & Integration

(26) Staff (*Dandasana*) - in a seated position stretch your legs out in front of you. Keep both your legs and your feet flexed (toes curling toward your face), lengthen out through your heels. Keep your torso upright and spine lengthened. You can rest your hands lightly on the floor under your shoulders or on your thighs. *Stay at least 5 complete breaths.*

(27) Cobbler (*Baddhakonasana*) - come to a seated position with the soles of your feet together, knees out to the side. Keep your back straight, spine lengthened. *Stay for 3 complete breaths.*

(28) Butterfly - while in Cobbler, move your feet forward 3-4", about a foot in front of your knees, keeping the soles together. Inhale fully and as you exhale fold the torso forward over your legs, forehead dropping toward your feet. You can round your back. Let your chin rest on your collarbone. Keep your arms, shoulders and neck completely relaxed. Let the body surrender into the pose continuing to let go of any holding and tension. As you exhale in the pose draw your lower belly in toward your spine and keep the belly drawn in. Practice Mindful Awareness, let go of thinking and stay connected to your body and breath. *Remain in the pose a minimum of 3 minutes.* With practice increase the time to 5 minutes.

(29) Cobbler - from Butterfly slowly come up to Cobbler. You can stretch your legs out in front of you and lean back with your weight on your hands placed on the floor behind your shoulders. *Rest for a few breaths.*

(30) Sphinx – start by lying down on your stomach, head turned to the side. Stay for 3 complete breaths, then rise up onto your elbows and forearms. Elbows placed directly under the shoulders, arms resting on the floor shoulder width apart, legs and buttocks relaxed. Put a little pressure into your forearms and elbows so the chest does not sag toward the floor. Keep the belly soft. Practice Mindful Awareness, let go of thinking and stay connected to your body and breath. *Remain in the pose a minimum of 3 minutes. With practice, increase the time to 5 minutes.*

(31 & 32) Resting to Full Body Twist - from lying on your stomach roll over onto your back resting for 5 complete breaths. Then bend your left leg and with your hands on your left knee, bring it toward your chest. Step the left foot over to the outside of the right knee or thigh. Reach your left arm out to the left side along the floor, back of left shoulder in contact with the floor. Holding your left knee with your right hand, inhale and as you exhale, gently pull the left knee over to the right, bent left leg crossing over the straight right leg. Keep the back of your shoulders against the floor. *Remain for 1 minute.* Then come to lying on your back and repeat the pose as described with your right leg (crossing it over to the left, right arm reaching out to the right side).

(33) Corpse (*Savasana*) - after completing the Full Body Twist remain on your back. Separate your feet shoulder width apart and let the legs and feet roll open. Bring your hands about a foot away from the side of your body, palms open toward the ceiling. Walk your shoulders down away from your ears. Pick your head up, lengthen your neck and settle the head again. Let your body settle into a deep state of relaxation. Allow any pressure or tension from the scalp, forehead, temples, jaw to release to the floor where the back of your head rests. Let your body be completely held by the floor. Let your awareness remain with your breathing. *Stay for at least 5 minutes.* This is a good time to practice Deep Relaxation Breathing. End *Savasana* completely relaxed, breathing naturally.

Simple Practice

Centering & Opening

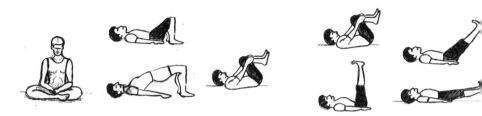

Opening (continued)

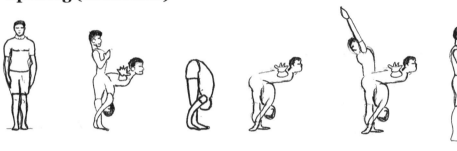

Resiliency

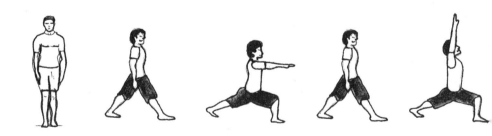

Closing & Integration

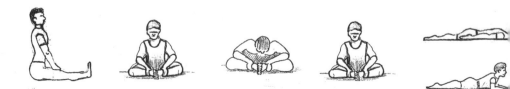

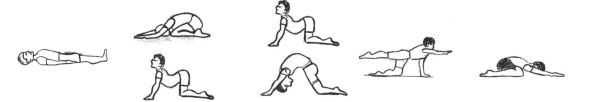

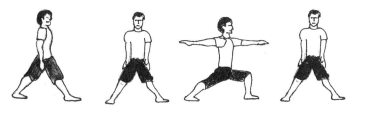

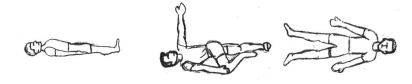

Chakras

Yoga and other transformational approaches for unifying mind, body and emotions to access the Divine Presence within oneself, incorporate the subtle energy system of *chakras* into their teachings and understandings. *Chakra* is a Sanskrit word for wheel. Although yoga teachings have greatly contributed to the understanding of *chakras* in modern times, there is a cross-cultural tradition of recognizing subtle energy centers in the body by various spiritual traditions. In early Christianity they were often referred to as "centers of the soul of man."

Chakras are energy centers in the body said to be perpetually rotating where prana or life force energy flows, collects and is distributed. *Chakras* function as fly-wheels to regulate the flow of energy throughout the body, to the mind and beyond. Yoga also acknowledges many channels in the body called *nadis* through which energy flows. The most important *nadi* in the body is the *sushumna nadi* inside the spinal column, the main channel for the flow of nervous energy. There are seven main *chakras* located along the *sushumna nadi* aligned in ascending order from the base of the spine to the crown of the head, though they may express themselves externally at various points of the body (below the navel, solar plexus, sternum, throat, forehead).

In relationship to *chakras* it is important to mention *kundalini* which is often misunderstood due to contradictory definitions of it. In yogic philosophy *kundalini* represents a coiled serpent lying dormant at the base of the spine. According to ancient texts on *kundalini* the serpent can be removed through *pranayama* and *asana* practices allowing for the free flow of *prana* up the *sushumna nadi,* piercing each *chakra* one-by-one, and bringing awakening to the practitioner.

1st Root Chakra
Sanskrit name: *Muladhara*
Location: base of spine
Symbol: gold cube
Represents: survival, connection with the earth, security, grounding

2nd Vital Force Chakra
Sanskrit name: *Svadhisthana*
Location: 2 inches below navel
Symbol: silver crescent
Represents: sense of worthiness, belonging, desire, sexuality, relationships

3rd Power Chakra
Sanskrit name: *Manipura*
Location: between the navel and solar plexis
Symbol: red inverted diamond
Represents: power center, will, seat of emotions

4th Heart Chakra
Sanskrit name: *Anahata*
Location: base of sternum
Symbol: blue six-pointed star
Represents: compassion and unconditional love

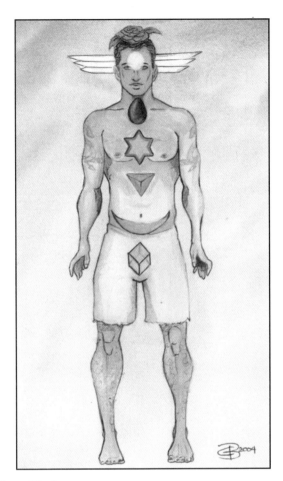

5th Communication Chakra
Sanskrit name: *Vishuddha*
Location: base of throat
Symbol: black onyx egg
Represents: communication, purity, center of expression and creativity

6th Third Eye Chakra
Sanskrit name: *Ajna*
Location: middle of forehead
Symbol: white-winged globe
Representss: intuition, understanding of life's lessons, clear insight

7th Crown Chakra
Sanskrit name: *Sahasrara*
Location: crown of head (at the top)
Symbol: red rose
Represents: awareness of union with the Source, connection with God, Enlightenment

Basic Practice

This is a well-structured and solid introduction to practicing many of the fundamental asanas of yoga. It is intended to provide a beginning and complete practice for anyone who is in reasonably good physical condition. It is recommended to do the Basic Practice regularly for at least six months before moving onto the Intermediate Practice.

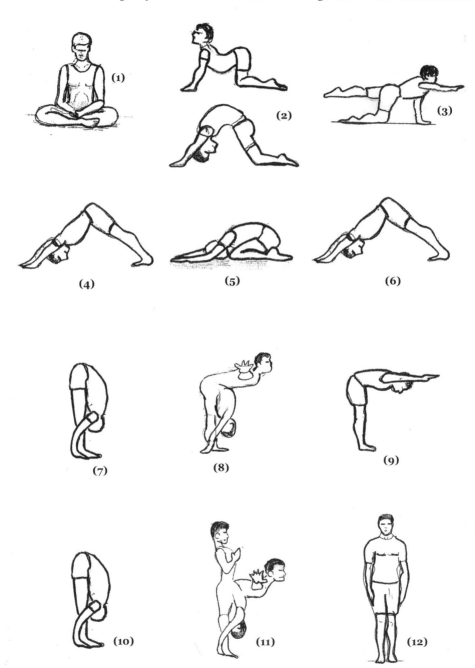

Centering & Opening

(1) Easy Pose (*Sukhasana*) – sit in cross-legged position, allow the spine to lengthen gently toward the crown of the head; chest open, shoulders relaxed. Chin dropped slightly toward the chest, head positioned so openings of ears are aligned with the shoulder joints. Shift weight slightly forward on sitting bones to create an arch in the lower back. Proper alignment assists in keeping the body stable and still, supporting meditation practice. If unable to sit in this position, you can sit on a chair or on a bunk with your back supported. *Sit quietly for 5 minutes (see Daily Meditation Practice or Expanding Awareness of Breath).*

(2) Cow/Cat – begin in Cow moving into the position on inhalation, allowing the back and spine to arch, tailbone tilted upward, arms straight with wrists under shoulders and knees under hips. Tilt head back and look up between eyebrows. Then as you exhale transition to Cat, rounding the spine and back, drawing the lower belly in toward the spine, tucking the tailbone between the legs, bringing your chin to the collarbone, looking to the tip of your nose. As your chin comes to your collarbone complete the exhale expelling all the air from the lungs. *Duration: 10 repetitions, inhaling slowly into Cow and exhaling slowly into Cat.*

(3) Sunbird (*Chakravakasana*) – start with wrists under shoulders, knees under hips. Reach your right arm straight out in front of you, and lift and extend your left leg straight back behind you. Arm and leg parallel to floor extending out through fingertips and toes. Then switch reaching forward with left arm and lifting the right leg. *Duration: 5 complete breaths each side, breathing slowly through the nose.*

(4) Downward Facing Dog (*Adhomukha Svanasana*) - starting with wrists under shoulders and knees under hips, hip width apart, walk your hands at least a hand length forward keeping them shoulder width apart and fingers spread wide. Curl your toes under and lift the body. Press your hands firmly into the floor extending your arms, shifting your chest toward your legs while allowing the spine to lengthen toward its base. Keep the back of your head in alignment with your arms. Legs are firmly flexed, no wider than hip width, heels press toward the floor. When first going into Down Dog you can bend one leg and straighten the opposite one, going back and forth, then finally straighten both legs and settle into pose. Heels will probably remain off floor. *Duration: 5 complete breaths.*

(5) Child's Pose (*Balasana*) – spread knees wide apart, drop buttocks toward feet settling sitting bones onto heels if possible. Keep the spine lengthened as you rest your forehead on the mat or a rolled up towel. Arms can be resting out in front of you or alongside your legs. *Duration: at least 10 complete, deep, relaxed breaths. Focus your attention on your forehead resting against the floor.*

(6) Downward Facing Dog – inhale up to Down Dog again. See alignment of body as described in (4) and focus on your exhalation as you exhale completely. *Duration: 5-10 complete breaths.*

(7) Standing Forward Fold (*Uttanasana*) – from Down Dog inhale walking your hands toward your feet, keeping your legs straight and hip width apart. When you come onto your feet, keep your weight evenly balanced from side to side and heel to toe. Legs stay flexed as you allow the torso to fold over the legs, spine lengthening toward the crown of your head. *Duration: 5 complete breaths*

(8 & 9) Standing Half Forward Fold (*Ardha Uttanasana*) – from Standing Forward Fold, on an inhale bring your back up parallel with the floor first spreading your arms out to the side, then lengthen your arms out in front of you. Arms, back of head and neck and spine all in parallel alignment. Keep your weight firmly balanced on your feet and extend your arms out through your fingertips. *Duration: 5 complete breaths*

(10) Standing Forward Fold – from Standing Half Forward Fold, on the fifth exhale fold forward again into the full Standing Forward Fold. Keep legs flexed, weight balanced on feet, spine lengthened, neck relaxed. *Duration: 5-10 complete breaths.*

(11) Transition to Standing/Mountain – from Standing Forward Fold inhale and come up to Half Forward Bend with arms stretched out to side parallel with floor. On next inhale continue raising the torso keeping the legs flexed and spine lengthened, sweeping the arms up from the sides of the body until the palms of the hands meet over head (see fig. 14). Look to your hands above your head, and as you exhale extend the arms out to the side and down, bringing your palms together and lifting them to your sternum (heart) in a prayer gesture. *Stay here for 5 complete breaths.*

(12) Mountain (*Tadasana*) – keeping your legs flexed, weight balanced on your feet, hip width apart, spine lengthened, shoulder blades slightly together and arms dangling along your side, close your eyes. Staying grounded through the soles of your feet, focus all of your awareness on the sensation of your breath moving in and out of the nose. *Duration: 5-10 complete breaths.*

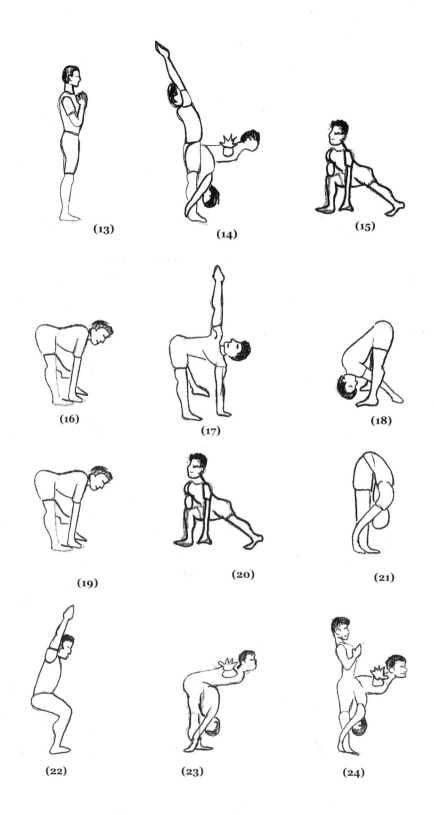

(13) (14) (15)

(16) (17) (18)

(19) (20) (21)

26 (22) (23) (24)

Opening (continued)

(13 & 14) Mountain to Standing Forward Fold – bring your hands together in front of your heart at your sternum. Pause for a breath or two. Then upon inhaling, sweep your arms out to the side raising them so that your hands come together over your head. Look to your hands, and upon exhaling, fold forward keeping the spine lengthened while sweeping the arms downward along side your body and settling into the forward fold for *2 complete breaths.*

(15) Low Lunge – from Standing Forward Fold bring your back up parallel with the floor and as you fold your torso forward, step your left leg and foot back into a lunge. This is a "runner's lunge" with the hips down, looking forward, chest open, hands on fingertips, lifting up behind the knee, back leg extends through the heel, stay on the ball of the foot. *Remain here for 3 complete breaths.*

(16) Standing Spread Leg (*Padottanasana*) – from the Low Lunge begin to move the upper body to the left, spinning and planting your left foot and as your body moves to the center, turning your right foot so your feet are in parallel alignment 4-5 feet apart. The hip joints should be aligned with the ankle joints. Place your hands or fingertips on the floor under your shoulders; lengthen your spine keeping it parallel with the floor. Back of the head and neck stay aligned with the spine as you look down slightly ahead of you at the floor. Keep the legs flexed and strong. *Duration: 3 complete breaths.*

(17) Standing Spread Leg Twist – while in Standing Spread Leg bring your right hand directly under your face, and while keeping your spine extended, inhale and twist the torso open to the left raising the left arm. Turn to look at your left hand; engage your neck muscles so your head does not droop toward the floor. Keep your legs flexed. *Stay for 3 complete breaths, before coming back to Standing Spread Leg,* replacing your hands under your shoulders. Take a breath, and then move the left hand in front of your face and as you inhale, sweep the right arm up twisting the torso open to the right and looking toward the right hand. *Stay on this side for 3 complete breaths before coming back to Standing Spread Leg (16).*

(18) Standing Spread Leg Forward Fold – from Standing Spread Leg (16), walk your hands and arms under your legs keeping them shoulder width apart. Keep your arms straight, palms planted on the floor. Try not to round your back keeping the spine extended toward the crown of your head. *Stay for 3 complete breaths before coming back to Standing Spread Leg.*

(19) Standing Spread Leg to (20) Low Lunge to (21) Standing Forward Fold – from Standing Spread Leg start to move your upper body toward your right foot while pivoting that foot forward. Spin onto the ball of your left foot as you transition back to the Low Lunge. Take a breath and then on your next exhale step the left foot forward, hip width apart from the right foot, lift your back up parallel with the floor keeping your fingertips under your shoulders touching the floor, then fold forward over your legs to come into the Standing Forward Fold. Keep your weight balanced on your feet and your legs flexed. *Stay here for 2 complete breaths.*

(22) Powerful Squat (*Utkatasana*) – from the Standing Forward Fold, with your feet hip width apart, bend your knees and drop your tailbone as if you were going to sit in a chair. Place your hands on your knees and inhaling sweep your arms up shoulder width apart while staying in the squat. Your tailbone should be 4-6 inches higher than your knees. Try to tuck the tailbone slightly as you extend your arms and ribcage upward. *Duration: 5 complete breaths.*

(23) Standing Forward Fold – from the Powerful Squat straighten your legs and fold the torso forward bringing your back parallel with the floor, arms stretched out to the side in Standing Half Forward Fold. Then exhale and fold forward into the Standing Forward Fold. *Duration: 5 complete breaths.*

(24) Transition to Standing/Mountain – from Standing Forward Fold inhale and come up to Half Forward Fold with arms stretched out to the side, parallel with floor. On the next inhale continue raising the torso keeping the legs flexed and spine lengthened, sweeping the arms up from the sides of the body until the palms of the hands meet over head. See figure (14). Look to your hands above your head, and as you exhale while standing, extend the arms out to the side and down, bringing your palms together and lifting them to your sternum (heart) in a prayer gesture. *Stay here for 5 complete breaths.*

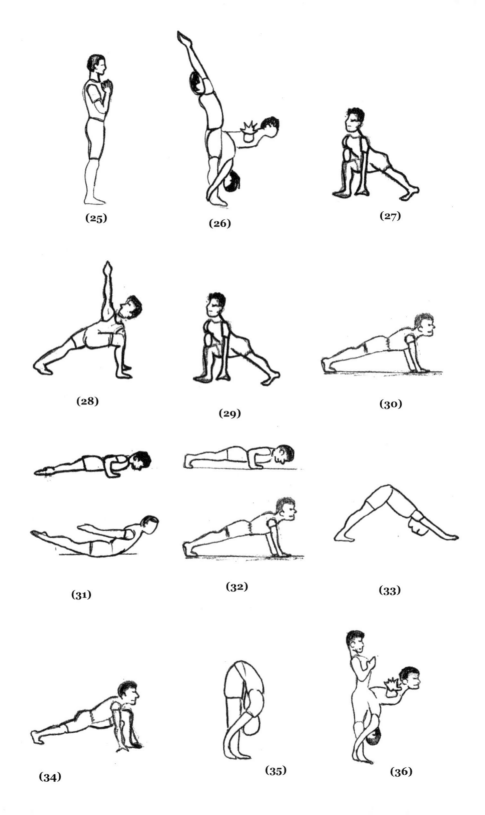

(25)   (26)   (27)

(28)   (29)   (30)

(31)   (32)   (33)

28

(34)   (35)   (36)

Purification

This series of the practice is called Sun Salutations (*Surya Namaskara*). It is to be practiced by going through the entire set from (25) to (36), addressing first one side of the body, then the other side. This means that for poses (27, 28 & 29), you do the first set with the left leg back, and for pose (34) with the left leg forward. For the second set you take the right leg back for poses (27, 28 & 29), and the right leg forward for pose (34). All the other poses are performed in both sets as illustrated and described.

(25 & 26) Mountain to Standing Forward Fold – see description (13 & 14).

(27) Low Lunge – see description (15), step the left foot and leg back.

(28) Lunge Twist – while in the Low Lunge place the left hand under the left shoulder and twist your torso open to the right. Extend your right arm and hand toward the ceiling. Keep the back leg straight, lifting up behind the knee. *Duration: 5 complete breaths.*

(29 & 30) Low Lunge to Plank – from the Lunge Twist bring your right arm down and come back into the Low Lunge for a breath. Then step the right leg back and come into Plank (push-up position). *Stay in Plank for 3 complete breaths.*

(31) Resting to Locust (*Salabhasana*) – from Plank come down onto the floor resting your forehead on the mat. Take a couple of breaths, then on your next exhale lift your head and chest, lift your legs and extend your arms back behind you with your palms facing. Keep your knees lifted, legs and feet close together and draw your shoulder blades together. Keep lifting up from the sternum. *Duration: 5 complete breaths.*

(32 & 33) Resting to Downward Facing Dog – from Locust come down onto the floor resting your forehead with your hands under your shoulders, staying for 2 breaths. Then curl your toes under and press up to Plank, and back to Downward Facing Dog. See description (4). *Stay in Down Dog for 3 complete breaths, exhaling completely out your nose.*

(34 & 35) Low Lunge to Standing Forward Fold – from Down Dog exhale and step the left foot forward into the Low Lunge, then step the right foot next to the left and bring your back up parallel with the floor. Try to keep your fingertips in touch with the mat; keep the legs flexed/straight. Inhale and as you exhale bend into the Standing Forward Fold. *Remain for 5 complete breaths.*

(36) Transition to Mountain – from Standing Forward Fold, inhale and come up to Mountain. See description (24). *Remain in Mountain for 2 complete breaths before starting the set over.*

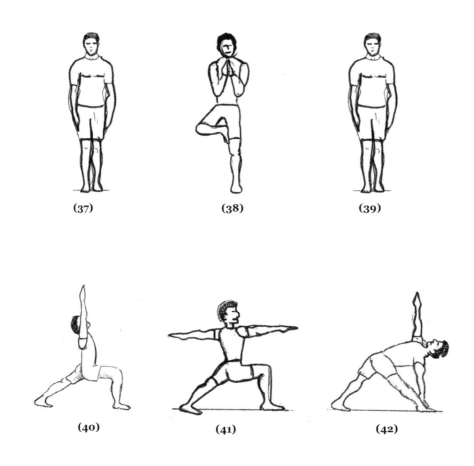

(37)   (38)   (39)

(40)   (41)   (42)

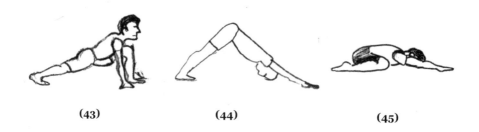

(43)   (44)   (45)

Resiliency

(37) Mountain (*Tadasana*) – stand in Mountain with arms by your side. *Take a few breaths feeling yourself balanced on both legs and feet.*

(38 & 39) Tree (*Vrksasana*) & Mountain – from Mountain shift your weight into your left leg. Feel yourself grounded through that flexed leg. When ready, pick up your right foot placing and pressing it to the inside of your left thigh, right heel as close to the left groin as possible. Keep your spine lengthened. Bring your hands together in front of your heart at the sternum. Find a spot on the floor to focus your gaze, breath easily. *Stay 5-10 complete breaths before stepping back to Mountain. Then repeat, this time lifting the left foot onto the inside of the right thigh.* Once you become accustomed to being in the pose you can raise your hands arms over your head, shoulder width apart, while staying balanced on the leg, then bring your hands back in front of your heart before stepping back into Mountain.

(40) Warrior I (*Virabhadrasana I*) – from Mountain step your left foot back 3-4 ft. planting its heel on the floor. Your front heel should be aligned with your back heel. Keep the back foot angled forward (45 to 60 degrees) so your hips can face forward. Inhale and raise your arms, and exhale bending the right leg as close to a 90 degree angle as possible. Your right knee should be directly over your right ankle. Keep the back leg straight and strong, back foot firmly rooted. The lower body sinks toward the floor while the upper body lengthens toward the ceiling. *Duration: at least 5 complete breaths. Then come back to Mountain and repeat on the other side (right leg back, left leg forward).*

(41) Warrior II (*Virabhadrasana II)* – from Mountain step your left foot back 4-5 ft. planting its heel firmly on the floor. Your front heel should be aligned with the middle of the arch of the back foot, the back foot angled slightly forward. Turn your hips to face the left side of the mat. Inhale and bring your arms up parallel with the floor and as you exhale bend the right leg as close to a 90 degree angle as possible. Your right knee should be directly over your right ankle. Keep the back leg straight lengthening it and pressing the back foot firmly into the mat. Look to the tips of your right fingers. Keep your torso vertically aligned over your hips. *Stay at least 5 complete breaths. Then come back to Mountain and repeat on the other side (right leg back, left leg forward).*

(42) Triangle (*Trikonasana*) - from Mountain step your left foot back 4-5 ft. planting its heel firmly on the floor. Your front heel should be aligned with the middle of the arch of the back foot, the back foot angled slightly forward. Turn your hips to face the left side of the mat. Inhale and raise your arms parallel with the floor, as you exhale reach as far forward as you can with your right arm parallel with the floor and shift your hips toward the back of the mat. Then place your left hand on your left hip and right hand on your right shin. Inhale and open the left side of your chest toward the ceiling, feeling the left hip stacking directly above the right hip as your torso and hips rotate open. When you are ready raise your left arm toward the ceiling and turn your head to look at your left hand. *Stay at least 5 complete breaths. Then come back to Mountain and repeat on the other side (right leg back, left leg forward).*

(43) Low Lunge – from Triangle sweep the raised hand forward, bending the front leg, placing your hands on either side of your front foot, and spinning onto the ball of the back foot to come into the Low Lunge.

(44) Downward Facing Dog – from the Low Lunge step back into Down Dog and *stay for 5 complete breaths.* Focus your attention on exhaling out the nose completely.

(45) Child's Pose – from Down Dog come up onto your toes and then drop your knees wide onto the edge of the mat. Bring your big toes together and settle into Child's Pose. See description (5). *Stay in Child's Pose at least 30 seconds.* Focus your attention on the sensation and weight of your forehead resting against the floor.

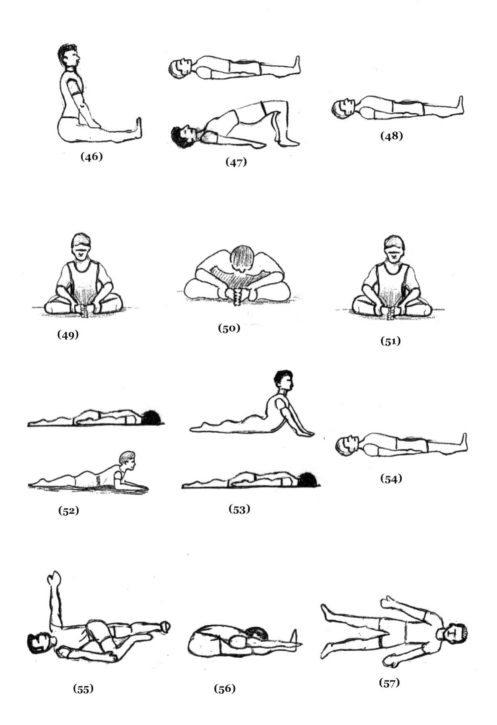

(46)   (47)   (48)

(49)   (50)   (51)

(52)   (53)   (54)

(55)   (56)   (57)

Closing & Integration

(46) Staff (*Dandasana*) – come to a seated position stretching your legs out in front of you while keeping your thighs flexed and spine lengthened. Lift up from the crown of your head and extend out through the heels of your flexed feet (toes curl toward your face). Place your hands under your shoulders on the floor or on your thighs. *Stay at least 5 complete breaths.*

(47 & 48) Bridge (*Setu Banda Sarvangasana*) – from Staff come lying down on your back. Bend your legs and walk your feet in close to your buttocks. You should be able to grab your heels with your fingers. Keeping your feet and knees hip with apart, press into the soles of your feet, lift from the lower belly and walk your shoulder blades in. Extend your arms along the floor. Keep pressing the feet into the floor engaging the muscles of the legs, buttocks and back to keep the body lifted. *Stay at least 5 breaths before rolling back down on your back.*

(49) Cobbler (*Baddhakonasana*) – beginning in Staff (46), bring the soles of your feet together, knees out to the side. Keep your back straight, spine lengthened. *Stay for 3 complete breaths.*
(50) Butterfly – while in Cobbler, move your feet forward 3-4" keeping the soles together. Inhale fully and as you exhale fold the torso forward over your legs, forehead dropping toward your feet. You can round your back. Keep your arms, shoulders and neck completely relaxed. Let the body surrender into the pose continuing to let go of any holding and tension. As you exhale in the pose draw your lower belly in toward your spine. Practice Mindful Awareness, let go of thinking and stay connected to your body and breath. *Remain in the pose a minimum of 3 minutes. With practice increase the time to 5 minutes.*
(51) Cobbler – from Butterfly slowly come up to Cobbler. Stretch your legs out in front of you and lean back with your weight on your hands placed on the floor behind your shoulders. *Rest for a few breaths.*

(52) Sphinx – start by lying down on your stomach, head turned to the side. *Stay for 3 complete breaths,* then rise up onto your elbows and forearms. Elbows placed directly under the shoulders, arms resting on the floor shoulder width apart, legs and buttocks relaxed. Put a little pressure into your forearms and elbows so the chest does not sag toward the floor. Keep the belly soft. Practice Mindful Awareness. *Remain in the pose a minimum of 3 minutes. With practice increase the time to 5 minutes or move into Seal (53) for the final 2 minutes.*

(53) Seal – after being in Sphinx for 3 minutes, press your palms into the floor and straighten your arms. Keep the legs and buttocks relaxed. Be careful not to force yourself to stay in the pose if it feels like too much pressure on the lower back. *Remain in Seal for 2 minutes before coming back down to Sphinx first before lying down and turning your head to the other side.*

(54 & 55) Resting to Full Body Twist (*Jathara Parivartanasana*) – from lying on your stomach roll over onto your back resting for 5 complete breaths. Then bend your left leg and with your hands on your left knee, bring it toward your chest. Step the left foot over to the outside of the right knee or thigh. Reach your left arm out to the left side along the floor, back of left shoulder in contact with the floor. Holding your left knee with your right hand, inhale and as you exhale, gently pull the left knee over to the right, bent left leg crossing over the straight right leg. Keep the back of your shoulders against the floor. *Remain for 1 minute. Then come to lying on your back and repeat the pose as described with your right leg (crossing it over to the left, right arm reaching out to the right side).*

(56) Seated Forward Fold (*Pachimottanasana*) – starting in Staff, see description (46), inhale reaching your arms up over your head and exhale folding your torso over your legs, grabbing your feet or your shins. Keep your legs and feet flexed, toes curling toward your face. Lengthen your spine to keep weight off your lower back. *Remain in pose 1 minute.*

(57) Corpse (*Savasana*) – after completing Seated Forward Fold, lie down on your back. Separate your feet shoulder width apart and let the legs and feet roll open. Bring your hands about a foot away from the side of your body, palms open toward the ceiling. Walk your shoulders down away from your ears. Pick your head up, lengthen your neck and settle the head again. Let your body settle into a deep state of relaxation. Allow any pressure or tension from the scalp, forehead, temples, jaw to release to the floor where the back of your head rests. Let your body be completely held by the floor. Let your awareness remain with your breathing. *Stay for at least 5 minutes.* This is a good time to practice Deep Relaxation Breathing (*Viloma Pranayama*). End *Savasana* completely relaxed breathing naturally.

Basic Practice

Centering & Opening

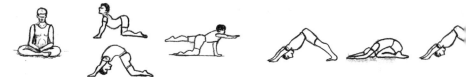

Opening (continued)

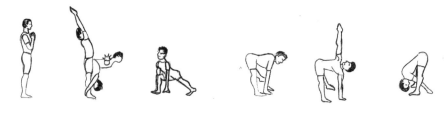

Purification

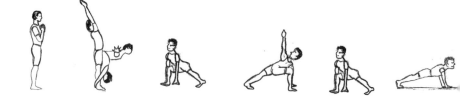

Resiliency

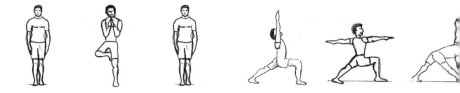

Closing & Integration

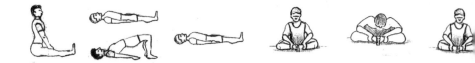

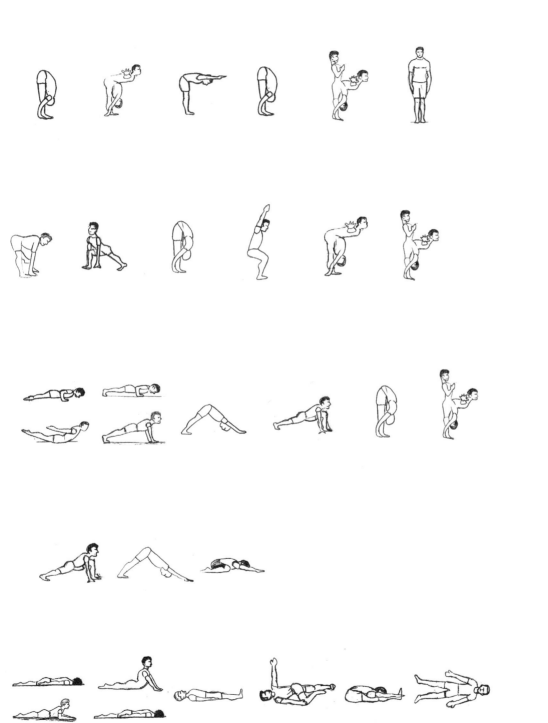

35

A Deeper Understanding of Yoga

In the West, the reasons for practicing yoga typically include: weight control, improved muscle tone, flexibility, coordination, stamina, restful sleep and inner well being. While these benefits are real and undeniable, they are entirely secondary to the traditional aim of yoga. Yoga seeks to cultivate a focused awareness of one's deepest being, one's True Self. The physical exercises augment the mental exercises that prepare the way for the transformation of consciousness and an intuitive experience of the divine.

Yoga involves a systemic approach to attaining the highest level of consciousness by unraveling the obstacles that stand in the way of being centered, rooted, sensitized to the presence of God within the human person. Seekers of conscious union with the divine in various ancient civilizations discovered that by keeping the body still you can calm the mind; that by concentrating your attention, you settle the body; and that by certain methods of breath-control, the mind becomes quiet and focused.

Yoga facilitates contemplative prayer by quieting the mind and cluing us into the mystery from which our being springs. The physical exercises (*asanas*) simply prepare the body and nervous system for the ensuing meditation. While yoga prepares one for meditation it is in itself meditation-in-motion. *Asanas* are correctly practiced only if they fulfill the central purpose of stilling the mind.

On the surface *asanas* look like a collection of stretching exercises coupled with breathing techniques, however the postures are to be performed with grace and control as a type of meditation. Their purpose is to bring one into a state of inner quiet, rebalancing the opposing forces within us to experience peace and inner harmony. As an example, during periods of stress when we experience discomfort in the neck, shoulders and back, the body is reacting to chronically stressed muscles. The first step to restoring inner peace is to relax the body. Stretching and lengthening muscles that are contracted helps to balance both the body and mind. What happens in the body affects the mind, just as the mind affects the body.

There are two aspects to the practice of *asanas*: the external form that works through the body, and the internal form that works through the mind. It is often popular to stress the external form, the technique, at the expense of the internal form, the attitude or intention. In reality the physical postures are the external vehicle for the more important "inner posture" – the experience of stillness within. This "inner posture" can be maintained even while the external posture is constantly changing.

Practicing *asanas* is a vehicle for inner awareness, and therefore a way to practice a different attitude toward everyday life. It is not unusual that internal attitudes and perceptions begin to change with the practice of yoga and meditation. Focusing on dispersing inner tension leads to acceptance, integration and peace. Experiencing inflexibility in the body can shed light on inflexible attitudes and states of mind. Postures can serve as a gateway for encountering limitations and fear. When you intentionally encounter bodily limitations and resistance from stiffness in muscles and joints, holding the postures becomes a powerful vehicle to explore where you are in the moment - mentally, emotionally and physically. The way to progress at that point is to accept your limitations, your condition, unconditionally.

In challenging life situations there are two divergent roads. You can say, "I've had enough of this; it is too difficult, uncomfortable and painful." In doing so you buy into limiting beliefs you hold about yourself and take refuge in regret, denial and/or escape activities. Or you can say, "Even though this is uncomfortable, difficult and painful, I'm going to face this and work through it." By "holding your posture," and releasing and relaxing into it as much as you can, you discover that you can actually extend beyond your preconceived limitations and fears.

Intermediate Practice

This represents a fairly challenging asana routine for those in sound physical condition. It is intended for a more experienced practitioner and comprises most of the fundamental yoga asanas, Unless you have done the Basic Practice for the prescribed period of time, the Intermediate Practice is not recommended as a starting asana practice.

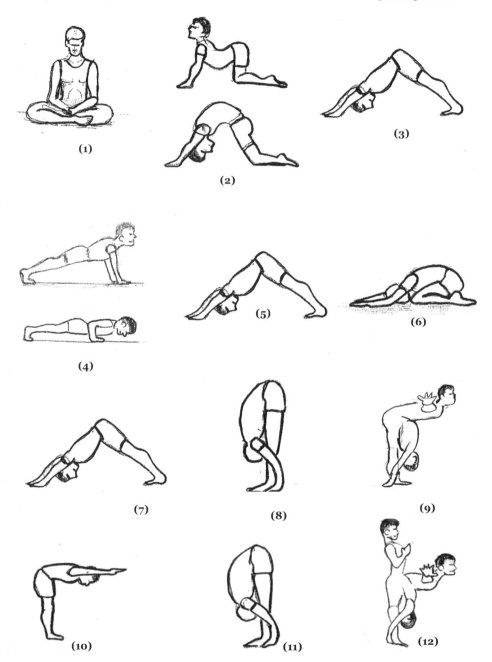

(1)

(2)

(3)

(4)

(5)

(6)

(7)

(8)

(9)

(10)

(11)

(12)

Centering & Opening

(1) Easy Pose (*Sukhasana*) – seated in cross-legged position. Allow the spine to lengthen gently toward the crown of the head; chest open, shoulders relaxed. Chin dropped slightly toward the chest, head positioned so openings of ears are aligned with the shoulder joints. Shift weight slightly forward on sitting bones to stabilize arch in the lower back. Proper alignment assists in keeping the body stable and still, supporting meditation practice. If unable to sit in this position, you can sit on a chair or a bunk with your back supported. *Sit quietly for 5 minutes.* (See Daily Meditation Practice or Expanding Awareness of Breath.)

(2) Cow/Cat – begin in Cow moving into position on inhalation, allowing the back and spine to arch, tailbone tilted upward, belly relaxed, arms straight with wrists under shoulders and knees under hips, hip width apart. Tilt head back looking up at eyebrows. Then as you exhale completely transition to Cat, rounding the spine and back, drawing the lower belly in toward the spine, tucking the tailbone between the legs, bringing your chin to the collarbone, looking to the tip of your nose. As your chin comes to your collarbone complete the exhale expelling all the air from the lungs. *Duration: 10 repetitions, inhaling slowly into Cow and exhaling slowly into Cat.*

(3) Downward Facing Dog (*Adhomukha Svanasana*) - starting with wrists under shoulders and knees under hips, walk your hands at least a hand length forward keeping them shoulder width apart and fingers spread wide. Curl your toes under and lift the body. Press your hands firmly into the floor extending your arms, shifting your chest toward your legs while allowing the spine to lengthen toward its base. Inner armpits open toward the floor. Keep the back of your head in alignment with your arms. Legs are firmly flexed, no wider than hip width, heels press toward the floor. When first going into Down Dog you can bend one leg and straighten the opposite one, going back and forth, then finally straighten both legs and settle into pose. Heels will probably remain off floor. *Duration: 5 complete breaths.*

(4 & 5) Plank to Chaturanga (*Chaturanga Dandasana*) to Downward Facing Dog – from Downward Dog come to Plank (push-up position). Inhale and bring your body a couple of inches off the floor (*Chaturanga Dandasana*) and exhale pressing back to Plank. Hands are placed under the shoulders, legs and abdominal muscles flexed. Do this slowly 5-10 times. Then from Plank, exhale and press back to Downward Dog again, *staying for 3-5 complete breaths.*
(6) Child's Pose (*Balasana*) – from Downward Dog spread your knees wide apart and come onto the mat. Drop the buttocks toward feet sitting on heels if possible. Keep the spine lengthened as you rest your forehead on the mat or a rolled up towel. Arms can be resting out in front of you or alongside your legs. *Duration: at least 10 complete, deep, relaxed breaths.*

(7) Downward Facing Dog – inhale and come up on your hands and kness and then up to Down Dog again. Work on alignment of body as described in (3) and focus your awareness on the exhalation as you exhale completely. *Duration: 5 complete breaths.*
(8) Standing Forward Fold (*Uttanasana*) – from Down Dog bend your knees and as you exhale hop your feet forward toward your hands. Straighten your legs, keep your feet hip width apart, bring your back up parallel with the floor, and then exhale folding the torso over the legs. Keep your thighs flexed with your weight evenly balanced on your feet from side to side and heel to toe, spine lengthening toward the crown of your head. *Duration: 5 complete breaths.*

(9 & 10) Standing Half Forward Fold (*Ardha Uttanasana*) – from Standing Forward Fold on an inhale bring your back up parallel with the floor, first spreading your arms out to the side, then lengthen your arms out in front of you. Arms, back of head and neck and spine all in parallel alignment. Keep your weight firmly balanced on your feet and extend your arms out through your fingertips. *Duration: 5 complete breaths*
(11) Standing Forward Fold – from Half Forward Fold on the fifth exhale fold forward again into the full Standing Forward Fold. Keep legs flexed, weight balanced on feet, spine lengthened, neck relaxed. *Duration: 5 complete breaths.*
(12) Transition to Standing/Mountain – from Standing Forward Fold inhale and come up to Half Forward Bend with arms stretched out to the side parallel with floor. On next inhale continue raising the torso, keeping the legs flexed and spine lengthened, sweeping the arms up from the sides of the body until the palms of the hands meet over head. (See figure 14). Look to your hands above your head, and as you exhale extend the arms out to the side and down, bringing your palms together and lifting them to your sternum (heart) in a prayer gesture. *Stay here for 5 complete breaths.*

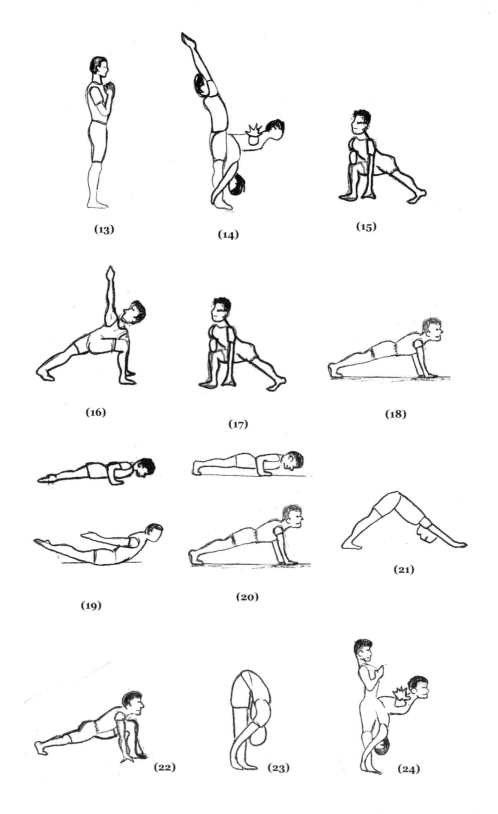

(13)

(14)

(15)

(16)

(17)

(18)

(19)

(20)

(21)

(22)

(23)

(24)

Purification

The following two series are variations of Sun Salutations (Surya Namaskara). They are to be practiced by going through each series individually, addressing first one side of the body and then the other side. This means that for the first series (13) to (24), you do the first set with the left leg back for poses (15, 16 & 17), and the left leg forward for pose (22). For the second set of the series you take the right leg back (15, 16 & 17), and the right leg forward for pose (22). All the other poses are performed in both sets as illustrated and described.

(13 & 14) Mountain (*Tadasana*) to Standing Forward Fold – start in Mountain with your hands together in front of your heart. Keeping your legs flexed, weight balanced on your feet, hip width apart, spine lengthened. After 2 complete breaths, on an inhale sweep your arms up out to the side, look at your hands as they come together over your head, and then exhale sweeping the arms out to the side toward the floor, folding the torso over the legs to come into the Standing Forward Fold. *Pause here for 2 breaths.*

(15) Low Lunge – from Standing Forward Fold inhale bringing your back up parallel with the floor and exhale as you fold your torso forward stepping your left leg and foot back into a "runner's lunge." Hips drop down, look forward, chest open, hands on fingertips, lifting up behind the knee, back leg extends through the heel, stay on the ball of the foot. *Remain here for 2 breaths.*

(16) Lunge Twist – while in the Low Lunge, place the left hand under the left shoulder and twist your torso open to the right and extend your right arm and hand toward the ceiling. Keep the back leg straight, lifting up behind the knee. *Duration: 5 complete breaths.*

(17 & 18) Low Lunge to Plank – from the Lunge Twist bring your right arm down and come back into the Low Lunge for a breath. Then step the right leg back and come into Plank (push-up position). *Stay in Plank for 2 complete breaths.*

(19) Locust (*Salabhasana*) – from Plank come down onto the floor resting your forehead on the mat. Take a couple of breaths, then on your next exhale lift your head and chest, lift your legs and extend your arms back behind you with your palms facing one another. Keep your knees lifted, legs and feet close and draw your shoulder blades together. Keep lifting up from the sternum. *Duration: 5 complete breaths.*

(20 & 21) Resting to Downward Facing Dog – from Locust come down onto the floor resting your forehead, staying for 2 breaths. Then curl your toes under and press up to Plank, and back to Down Dog, see description (3). *Stay in Down Dog for 3 complete breaths, exhaling completely out your nose.*

(22 & 23) Low Lunge to Standing Forward Fold – from Down Dog exhale and step the left foot forward into the Low Lunge, then step the right foot next to the left and bring your back up parallel with the floor. Try to keep your fingertips in touch with the mat; keep the legs flexed/straight. Inhale and as you exhale bend into the Standing Forward Fold. *Remain for 3 complete breaths.*

(24) Transition to Mountain – from Standing Forward Fold, inhale and come up to Mountain. See description for (12). *Remain in Mountain for 3 complete breaths before starting the set over.*

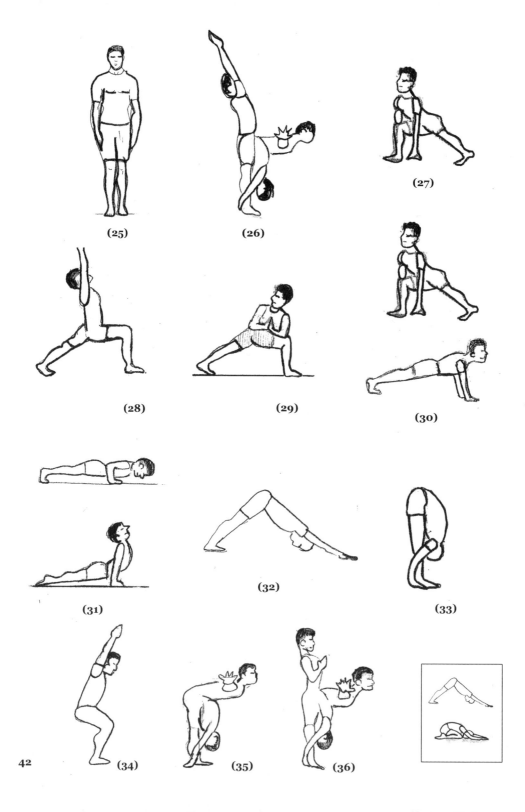

(25)　　　　　(26)

(27)

(28)　　　　　(29)

(30)

(31)

(32)

(33)

42　　(34)　　　(35)　　　(36)

Purification (continued)

For this second series (25) to (36) of Sun Salutations, you do the first set with the left leg back for (27, 28, 29 & 30), and the second set with the right leg back for those poses. The other poses are performed in both sets as illustrated and described.

(25 & 26) Mountain (*Tadasana*) to Standing Forward Fold – see description for 13 & 14. *Pause here for 2 breaths.*

(27) Low Lunge – see description for 15. *Stay here for 2 breaths.*

(28) Crescent Lunge (*Alanasana*) – from the Low Lunge place your hands on your right knee, then inhale and sweep your arms up over your head shoulder width apart. Keep the back leg straight lifting up behind the knee. Stay on the ball of the back foot extending through the heel. *Stay 5 complete breaths.*

(29) Revolved Lunge (*Parivrtta Parsvakonasana*) – from Crescent Lunge exhale and place the left elbow behind the right knee, bringing your hands together in front of your chest fingertips pointing up. Use the left elbow to help you twist the torso as you draw your right shoulder open. Keep the back leg straight lifting up behind the knee. Stay on the ball of the back foot extending through the heel. *Duration: 5 complete breaths.*

(30) Low Lunge to Plank – from Revolved Lunge inhale and take your left elbow off the right leg, and turning the torso forward place your fingertips down and come back into the Low Lunge for a breath. Then step the right leg back and come into Plank (push-up position). *Stay in Plank for 2 complete breaths.*

(31) Chaturanga Dandasana to Upward Facing Dog (*Urdhvamukha Svanasana*) – from Plank come down a couple of inches off the floor to *Chaturanga Dandasana*, then shift the chest and head forward while pressing upward to come into Upward Facing Dog. Lengthen the arms pressing the palms firmly into the floor under the shoulders. Lift from the crown of the head. Legs are flexed with knees off the floor, weight on the top of the feet, spine lengthening, look forward and slightly upward. *Stay 3-5 complete breaths.*

(32) Downward Facing Dog – from Upward Facing Dog shift onto the balls of your feet and *exhale back to Downward Facing Dog for 3 breaths.*

(33) Standing Forward Fold – from Down Dog bend your knees and as you exhale hop your feet forward toward your hands and come into Standing Forward Fold. See description for (8). *Stay for 3 breaths.*

(34) Powerful Squat (*Utkatasana*) – from the Standing Forward Fold, with your feet hip width apart, bend your knees and drop your tailbone as if you were going to sit in a chair. Place your hands on your knees and inhaling sweep your arms up shoulder width apart while staying in the squat. Your tailbone should be 4-6 inches higher than your knees. Try to tuck the tailbone slightly as you extend your arms and ribcage upward. *Duration: 5 complete breaths.*

(35) Standing Forward Fold – from the Powerful Squat straighten your legs and bring your back parallel with the floor, arms out to the side to Standing Half Forward Fold, then exhale folding forward into the Standing Forward Fold. *Duration: 5 complete breaths.*

(36) Transition to Mountain – from Standing Forward Fold, inhale and come up to Mountain. (See description figure 12). *Remain in Mountain for 3 complete breaths before starting the set over.*

Note: When you complete the second set rather than going from Standing Forward Fold (35) transitioning to Mountain Pose (36), go from Standing Forward Fold to Downward Facing Dog to Child's Pose. See description for (6). *Rest in Child's Pose for 10 complete breaths.*

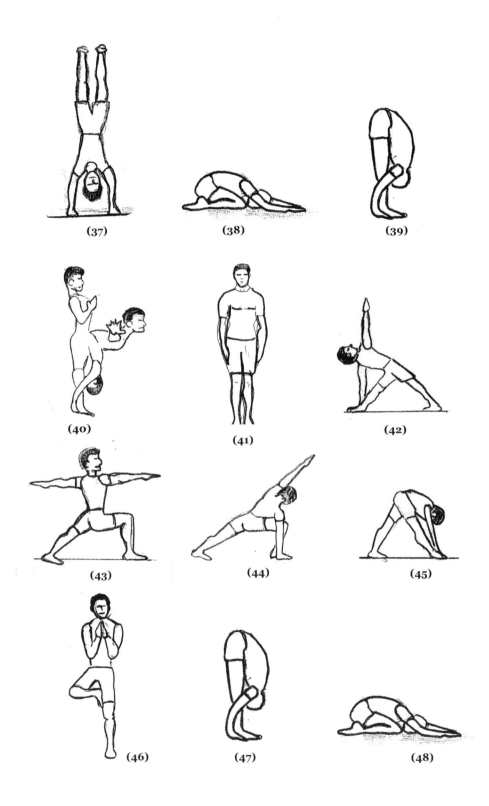

(37)   (38)   (39)

(40)   (41)   (42)

(43)   (44)   (45)

(46)   (47)   (48)

Resiliency

(37) Handstand – get into a Low Lunge position, see description (15), facing a wall or the inside of a cell door. Place your hands shoulder width apart about 9-12 inches away from the wall. If you are right handed, your right leg should be extended back in a Low Lunge. If you are left handed, your left leg back. Whatever feels most natural to kick up into a handstand against the wall. Kick the back leg up balancing your weight on your hands a couple of times getting used to the sensation. When you are ready, go all the way up. Once in a handstand your feet should be close together against the wall. Keep lengthening your arms, hands under your shoulders not wider. Keep looking toward the wall. Experiment with taking your feet off the wall to come into a balanced Handstand. *Try to hold the Handstand for 30 seconds, increasing to 1 minute with practice.*
(38) Child's Pose – see description (6). Come down from Handstand to Child's Pose *for 1 minute.*
(39) Standing Forward Fold – see description (8). From Child's Pose come to Standing Forward Fold for *5 complete breaths.*

(40 & 41) Transition to Mountain – see description (12). Remain for *3 complete breaths.*
(42) Triangle (*Trikonasana*) - from Mountain step your left foot back 4-5 ft. planting the heel firmly. Your front heel should be aligned with the middle of the arch of the back foot, the back foot angled slightly forward. Turn your hips to face left. Inhale and raise your arms parallel with the floor and as you exhale reach as far forward as you can with your right arm parallel with the floor while shifting your hips. Then place your left hand on your left hip and right hand on your right shin. Inhale and spin open the left side of your chest toward the ceiling. Feel the left hip stacking directly above the right hip as your torso and hips rotate open. When you are ready, raise your left arm toward the ceiling and turn your head to look at your left hand. *Stay at least 30 seconds.* Then come back to Mountain (41) and repeat on the other side (right leg back, left leg forward).

(43) Warrior II (*Virabhadrasana II*) - from Mountain step your left foot back 4-5 ft. planting the heel firmly. Your front heel should be aligned with the middle of the arch of the back foot, the back foot angled slightly forward. Turn your hips to face the left. Inhale and bring your arms up parallel with the floor, and as you exhale bend the right leg as close to a 90 degree angle as possible. Your right knee should be directly over your right ankle. Keep the back leg straight lengthening it and pressing the back foot down firmly. Look to the tips of your right fingers. Keep your torso vertically aligned over your hips. *Stay at 30 seconds. Then come back to Mountain (41) and repeat on the other side (right leg back, left leg forward).*
(44) Extended Side Angle (*Parsvakonasana*) – begin in Warrior II, see description (43), with your left leg and foot back. Stay in Warrior II for 3 complete breaths. Then place your left hand on your left hip and your right fingertips to the outside of your right foot (if this is too difficult you can place your right forearm on the top of your right thigh). Right leg is bent at a 90 degree angle. Rotate the left side of your chest and torso open and extend your left arm over your ear reaching out over the bent right leg. Your left arm should be a diagonal extension of your left leg. *Stay at least 30 seconds. Then repeat on the other side (right leg back, left leg forward).*
(45) Intense Side Stretch (*Parsvottanasana*) – begin standing in Mountain (41). Step your left foot back 3-4 ft. keeping the foot facing forward. Align the front right heel with the back left heel. Turn your hips to face forward. Place your hands on your hips and keeping your legs flexed and straight, bend forward from the waist bringing your back parallel with the floor. Then extend your arms forward over the right leg and as you exhale, fold the torso over the right leg, bringing your hands onto the floor on either side of the right foot or onto your shin. *Stay for 5 complete breaths. Then come back to Mountain and repeat on the other side (right leg back, left leg forward).*

(46) Tree (*Vrksasana*) - from Mountain (41) shift your weight into your left leg. Feel yourself grounded through that flexed leg. When ready, pick up your right foot placing and pressing it to the inside of your left thigh, right heel as close to the left groin as possible. Keep your spine lengthened. Bring your hands together in front of your heart at the sternum. Find a spot on the floor to focus your gaze, breathe easily. *Stay at least 5 complete breaths before stepping back to Mountain. Then repeat, this time lifting the left foot onto the inside of the right thigh.* Once you become accustomed to being in the pose you can raise your hands arms over your head, shoulder width apart, while staying balanced on the leg. Bring your hands back in front of your heart before stepping back into Mountain.
(47) Standing Forward Fold – see description (8). *Stay in Standing Forward Fold at least 5 complete breaths.*
(48) Child's Pose – see description (6). *Stay at least 10 complete breaths.*

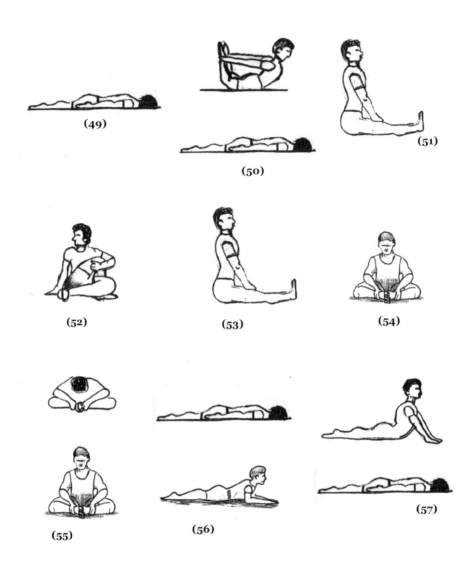

(49)

(50)

(51)

(52)

(53)

(54)

(55)

(56)

(57)

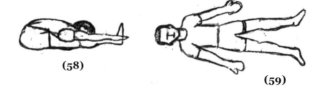

(58)

(59)

Closing & Integration

(49) Lying On Stomach – from Child's Pose (48), come lying down onto your stomach on the floor with your arms along side your body. Turn your head to the side. *Stay here a couple of breaths.*

(50) Bow (*Dhanurasana*) – while lying on your belly pick your head up and bend one leg at a time stretching your arms back to hold your ankles. On the next inhale pull on shins of the legs and raise the knees while at the same time lifting your chest and head. The arms and hands act like a bow to tighten and bend the body. Keep your knees and ankles hip width apart while you keep lifting. *Stay for 5 complete breaths or 30 seconds. Then release the ankles and bring the legs, chest and head back to the floor to relax an equal amount of time. Repeat the pose at least once again.*

(51) Staff Pose (*Dandasana*) – come to a seated position stretching your legs out in front of you while keeping the thighs flexed and the spine lengthened. Lift up from the crown of your head and extend out through the heels of your flexed feet (toes curl toward your face). Place your hands under your shoulders on the floor or on your thighs. *Remain for 5 complete breaths.*

(52) Seated Twist (*Ardha Matsyendrasana*) – from Staff Pose, bend the right leg placing your right heel on the floor, and bend the left leg allowing it to remain on the floor, left knee facing forward. Bring the left heel over to the outside of the right buttock. If possible, pick up the right leg and foot, crossing it over the left leg. See if you can place the outside of the right ankle up against the top of the left thigh as you plant the right foot on the floor. Bring your right hand directly behind your back close to your body to help keep the spine straight. Wrap the inner left elbow around the right knee. As you inhale, lengthen your spine, as you exhale twist the entire torso to the right. Look behind you over your opened right shoulder. *Stay for 10 complete breaths before switching your legs and twisting to the other side.*

(53) Staff Pose – *come back to Staff Pose for 5 breaths.*

(54) Cobbler (*Baddhakonasana*) – from Staff Pose bring the soles of your feet together, knees out to the side. Keep your back straight, spine lengthened. *Stay for 3 complete breaths.*

(55) Butterfly to Cobbler– while in Cobbler, move your feet forward 3-4" keeping the soles together. Inhale fully and as you exhale fold the torso forward over your legs, forehead dropping toward your feet. You can round your back. Keep your arms, shoulders and neck completely relaxed. Let the body surrender into the pose continuing to let go of any holding and tension. As you exhale in the pose draw your lower belly in toward your spine. Practice Mindful Awareness, let go of thinking and stay connected to your body and breath. *Remain in the pose a minimum of 3 minutes; with practice increase the time to 5 minutes.* From Butterfly slowly come up to Cobbler. Stretch your legs out in front of you and lean back with your weight on your hands placed on the floor behind your shoulders. *Rest for a few breaths.*

(56) Resting to Sphinx – start by lying down on your stomach, head turned to the side. *Stay for 3 complete breaths, then rise up onto your elbows and forearms.* Elbows placed directly under the shoulders, arms resting on the floor, shoulder width apart, legs and buttocks relaxed. Put a little pressure into your forearms and elbows so the chest does not sag toward the floor. Keep the belly soft. Practice Mindful Awareness, let go of thinking and stay connected to your body and breath. *Remain in the pose a minimum of 3 minutes. With practice increase the time to 5 minutes or move into Seal for the final 2 minutes.*

(57) Seal to Resting – after being in Sphinx for 3 minutes, press your palms into the floor and straighten your arms. Keep the legs and buttocks relaxed. Be careful not to force yourself to stay in the pose if it feels like too much pressure on the lower back. *Remain in Seal for 2 minutes before coming back down to Sphinx, and then lying down with your head turned to the side. Rest for 30 seconds.*

(58) Seated Forward Fold (*Pachimottanasana*) – starting in Staff Pose, see description (51), inhale reaching your arms up over your head and exhale folding your torso over your legs, grabbing your feet or your shins. Keep your legs and feet flexed, toes curling toward your face. Lengthen your spine to keep weight off your lower back. *Remain in pose 1 minute.*

(59) Corpse (*Savasana*) – after completing Seated Forward Fold, lie down on your back. Separate your feet shoulder width apart and let the legs and feet roll open. Bring your hands about a foot away from the side of your body, palms open toward the ceiling. Walk your shoulders down away from your ears. Pick your head up, lengthen your neck and settle the head again. Let your body settle into a deep state of relaxation. Allow any pressure or tension from the scalp, forehead, temples, jaw to release to the floor where the back of your head rests. Let your body completely surrender into the floor. Let your awareness remain with your breathing. *Stay for at least 5 minutes. This is a good time to practice Deep Relaxation Breathing (Viloma Pranayama). End Savasana completely relaxed breathing naturally.*

Intermediate Practice

Centering & Opening

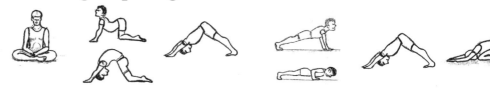

Purification

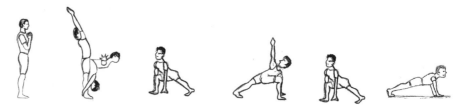

Purification (continued)

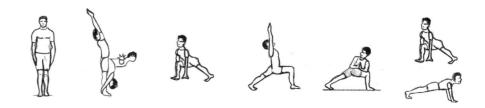

Resiliency

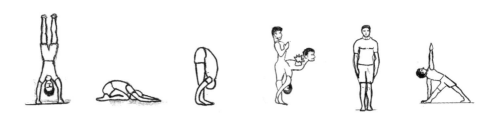

Closing & Integration

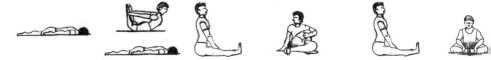

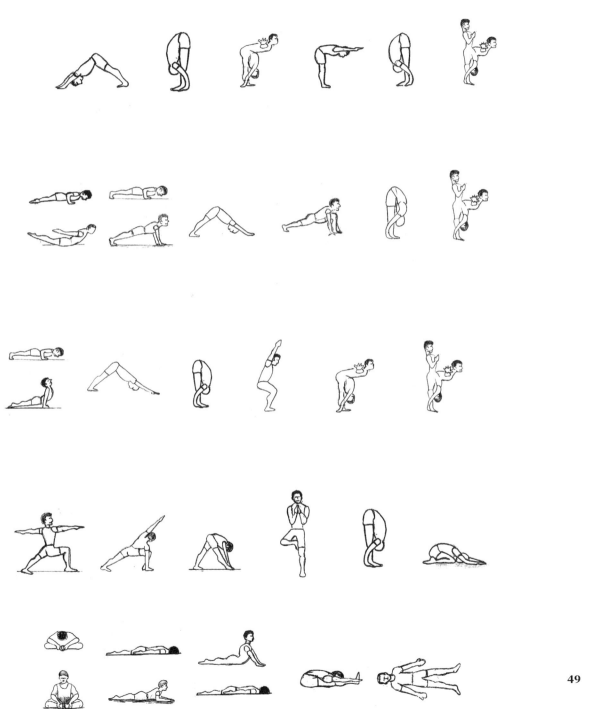

49

Self Image and the Imagined Self

It's seldom that we go through an hour or a day and not experience feelings of self-consciousness, tension, anger, depression, fear, sadness and envy. It is also common that during the course of a day, we experience pleasant states that we wish we had more often or would last forever. Trying to hide from negative states, to distract ourselves or run away, simply invites them to come back. Yet somehow the mind wants to convince itself that it only wants pleasant states.

The judging mind has an opinion about everything. It's full of noise and old learning. It is a mind imprisoned, addicted to maintaining an image of itself and always trying to be somebody.

It's very difficult to see what really is when we're actively filtering all input. The imaginary "I" is constantly and compulsively defining itself, and building an image of itself from passing thoughts. We select from the great mix of our experiences an image here and there, and discredit the rest through some sort of rationalization. We tend to judge and comment on everything from the point of view of the self-image of the moment. We become our states of mind rather than allowing them to just pass through.

When we open our minds and our hearts, not trying to understand, we allow the knowing mind to arise. Wisdom occurs in the mind that rests in not knowing, the still mind that simply is. In letting go of who we imagine ourselves to be, letting go of our thinking and attempts to control the world, we come upon our natural being that has been waiting patiently for us to come home. By gently letting go of everything, not by force but by seeing it all as a process and flow, we let go of being anyone and open to natural understanding that allows everything to come and go as it does.

Excerpt from *A Gradual Awakening*, by Stephen Levine, Random House, Inc.

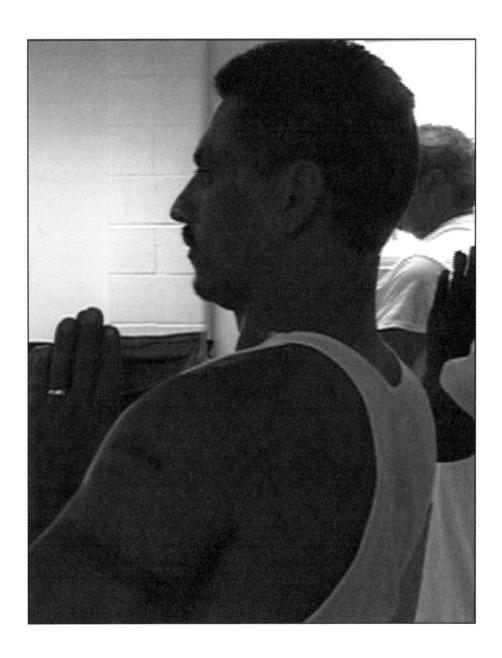

Two Levels of Perception

An important topic covered in the Yoga Sutra (*see page 3*) has to do with the way we perceive things. In the Sutra, Patanjali states there are two levels of perception:

AVIDYA - superficial perception, that literally means "incorrect comprehension" or misperception.
VIDYA - perception that is deeply rooted within us, and means "correct or clear understanding."

Avidya represents how the mind constantly misunderstands, misperceives or misinterprets people, situations and events causing us ongoing personal difficulties and suffering. As a result of these continuing misperceptions, we develop unconscious, habitual actions or reactions to events causing ourselves and others suffering. We take action only to find out later that we were mistaken. This habitual unconscious misperception and resulting behavior is called *samskara*. "Stuck on the wheel of *samskara*" is a term that is used to describe the repetitive cycle of personal disappointment and suffering we experience.

Avidya is fed by:

• Selfishness: ego; I am right.
• Desire: demands; I want. I deserve.
• Hate: rejecting people, ideas, etc. based on not being open.
• Fear: doubts about ourselves and concerns for other people's judgments.

Vidya is the opposite of *avidya* and represents correct or clear understanding, which results from a deep understanding within us that is not obscured by false perception. *Vidya* stems from clarity, and when experienced usually results in skillful action and things going well for us.

One of the goals of yoga is to reduce *avidya* and increase *vidya*. Yoga offers the opportunity to direct the mind without distraction. It provides a disciplined practice for the mind to pay close attention to thoughts, emotions and sensations in the body, thereby fostering self-awareness and an increased moment-to-moment consciousness. This can help break free of *smaskara* by decreasing misperceptions (*avidya*) so that true understanding (*vidya*) can take place.

Taoist Yoga

Taoism (also known as Daoism) refers to a Chinese philosophical tradition that has influenced Eastern Asia for over 2,000 years and in more recent times the western world with the introduction of yoga, martial arts and other Asian practices. *Tao* means "the path," "the way," or "the flow of the universe." Taoist practices seek to exercise the path of least resistance. Taoist philosophy emphasizes naturalness, vitality, peace, non-action ('effortless effort'), emptiness, detachment, flexibility, receptiveness and spontaneity as ways of guiding human behavior. The so-called three jewels of *Tao* are compassion, moderation and humility.

Taoist Yoga has its origins in the ancient *Dao Yin* stretching and static posture exercises that were practiced in Chinese Taoist monasteries as early as 200 B.C. Its physical practice, which is combined with breath work, as well as its overall intention, have obvious parallels to the classical Indian yoga that is presented throughout this book. The traditional goal of Taoist Yoga is to bring the mind and body into harmony for self-healing and spiritual development. Taoist Yoga also has some similarity to *Qigong* (*Chi Kung*). Both practices have similar roots and are based on the Taoist theory of nurturing and increasing the flow vital life force energy, or *chi/prana*, in the body for improved health, healing and overall well-being.

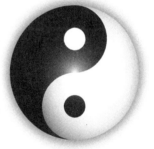

According to Taoist philosophy, *yin* and *yang* are opposite yet interconnected forces in the natural world. The concept of *yin* and *yang* serve as a primary guide for traditional Chinese medicine, various forms of martial arts, *Qigong* and Taoist Yoga. From a Taoist perspective *yang* energy is considered assertive by nature; *yin* is receptive. In yoga, strength oriented postures are typically *yang*, whereas gentler postures are *yin*. *Yang* poses exercise muscles and bones, whereas *yin* poses target joints, ligaments, tendons and connective tissue promoting the flow of *chi* to the organs of the body. It is important to include a mix of *yang* and *yin* poses to create balance in an *asana* practice. Additionally, each pose (*asana*) whether *yang* or *yin* presents the opportunity to express both forces of energy. In an assertive *yang* pose such as Downward Dog (*Adhoumukha Svanasana*), muscles and bones in the body are exerted, yet it is important to apply *yin* receptive energy by softening internally and keeping the breath flowing smoothly while holding the pose. In a *yin* pose, such as Butterfly, although the body is held in a receptive or somewhat passive posture, *yang* energy is asserted to draw the muscles of the lower belly in toward the spine and develop the mental and physical stamina required to hold the pose for an extended period of time.

Taoist Yoga circulates what is stagnant and calms what is agitated – harmonizing, stabilizing and rejuvenating the energy body. *Yang* element promotes the overall flow of life force energy, enhancing *chi* and removing blockages. *Yin* element promotes a contemplative stillness bringing awareness to present sensations, emotions and mind states.

Warrior Practice

The Warrior Practice is a unique, intermediate asana practice that combines influences of classical Raja Yoga with the martial arts-like movements of Taoist Yoga. It is intended for a more experienced and well-conditioned practitioner. It is recommended that one should have experience with the Intermediate Practice before moving onto the Warrior Practice. The Warrior Practice as described should take 90 minutes or slightly longer to complete.

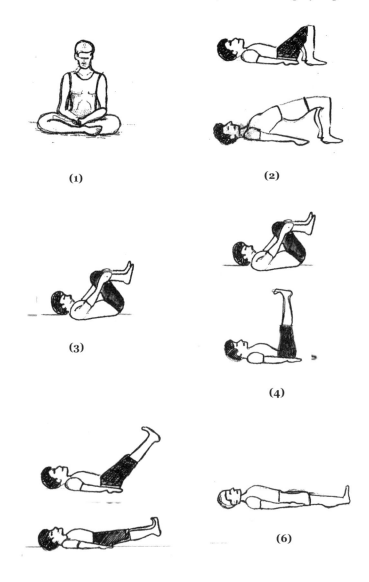

(1)

(2)

(3)

(4)

(5)

(6)

Centering & Opening

(1) Easy Pose (*Sukhasana*) - seated in cross-legged position, allow the spine to lengthen gently toward the crown of the head; chest open, shoulders relaxed. Chin dropped slightly toward the chest, head positioned so openings of ears are aligned with the shoulder joints. Shift weight slightly forward on sitting bones to stabilize arch in the lower back. Proper alignment assists in keeping the body stable and still, supporting meditation practice. If unable to sit in this position, you can sit on a chair with your back supported. *Sit quietly for 5 minutes* (see Daily Meditation Practice or Expanding Awareness of Breath).

(2) Bridge (*Setu Banda Sarvangasana*) - come lying down on your back. Extend your arms along side your body. Bend your legs and walk your feet in close to your buttocks. Keeping your feet and knees hip width apart. Inhale and lift the hips and buttocks pressing the soles of your feet into the floor. As you exhale, slowly roll the spine down one vertebra at a time. Continue moving with your breath, rising on inhale, lowering on exhale. After 5-6 repetitions, rise up into the bridge, walk your shoulder blades in toward one another, press your arms against the floor and stay in the pose. Keep pressing the feet into the floor engaging the muscles of the legs, buttocks and back to keep the body lifted. *Stay at least 5 complete breaths before rolling back down on your back.*

NOTE: *poses 3-6 are done as a continuous set.*

(3) Knees to Chest (*Apanasana*) - staying on your back lift your feet off the floor. With your arms extended, hold onto your knees (shoulder width apart) or upper shins. Inhale fully and as you exhale completely out your nose, draw your knees into your chest. *Repeat at least 3-4 times.*

(4) Legs 90° to Floor - after exhaling and drawing your knees toward your chest, inhale and raise your legs perpendicular (90°) to the floor, feet together. Keep your quadriceps muscles and feet flexed, toes curling toward your shins as you extend the heels toward the ceiling. Exhale completely as you draw your knees in to your chest. *Repeat 3-4 times.*

(5) Abdominal/Core Strength Building - from your legs raised 90° to the floor with feet together, lower the legs halfway to the floor (from 90° to 45°). Keep the legs and feet flexed as you extend out through your heels. Hold to the count of 10 before lowering the heels about 3-4 inches off the floor. Keeping the legs/heels lifted off the floor, inhale and take the legs wide apart; as you exhale bring them together. *10 repetitions.*

(6) Resting - after bringing your feet together on the last rep, slowly lower the heels to the floor. Separate your feet hip width apart; rest your hands on your lower belly below the navel. Let your legs and feet roll open. Pick you head up and lengthen your neck tucking your chin toward your chest before resting the back of the head on the mat. Feel your belly rising and falling under your hands with each breath, let yourself relax completely, keeping your awareness on your breathing rather than thoughts.
Stay for 5-10 breaths.

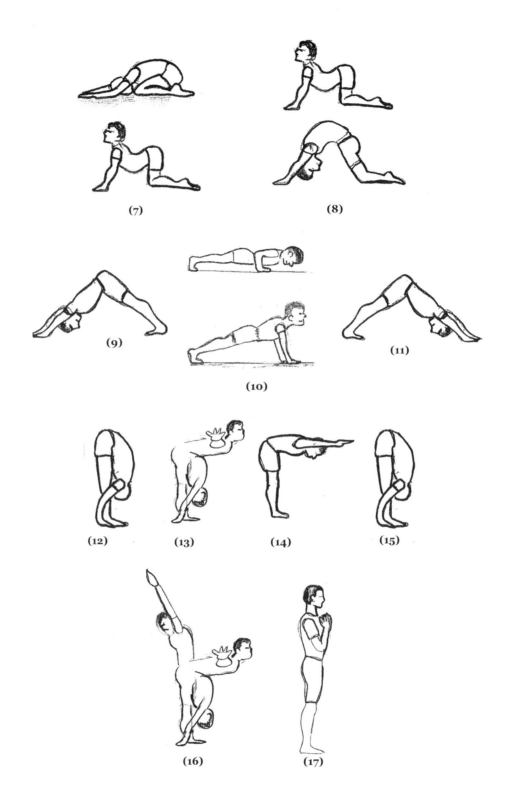

(7)

(8)

(9)

(10)

(11)

(12)

(13)

(14)

(15)

(16)

(17)

Opening (continued)

NOTE: *Poses 7-8 are done as a continuous set.*

(7) Child's Pose (*Balasana*) to Cow - spread knees hip width apart and sit back toward your heels with your arms out in front of you. Keep the spine lengthened as you rest your forehead on the mat. Inhale and slowly begin to rise onto your hands and knees letting your head be the last part of the body that comes up into Cow pose. Allow your back and spine to arch, tale bone tilted upward, belly relaxed, arms straight with wrists under shoulders and knees under hips. Tilt head back looking up toward eyebrows. As you exhale, slowly come back to Child's Pose, letting your head be the last part of your body that comes down as you look toward the tip of your nose. Continue moving back and forth from Child's Pose to Cow (*4-5 repetitions*), always moving with inhale and exhale as described.

(8) Cow/Cat - from Cow, rather than going back to Child's pose, as you exhale transition to Cat, rounding the spine and back, drawing the lower belly in toward the spine, tucking the tailbone between the legs, bringing your chin to the collarbone, looking to the tip of your nose. As your chin comes to your collarbone complete the exhale expelling all the air from the lungs. *4-5 repetitions.*

(9) Downward Facing Dog (*Adhomukha Svanasana*) - from Cow pose with wrists under shoulders and knees under hips, walk your hands at least a hand length forward keeping them shoulder width apart and fingers spread wide. Curl your toes under and lift the body. Press your hands firmly into the floor extending your arms, allowing the spine to lengthen toward its base, ribs lifting toward the hips. Keep the back of your head in alignment with your arms. Legs are firmly engaged/flexed, no wider than hip width, heels press toward the floor. When first going into Down Dog you can bend one leg and straighten the opposite one, going back and forth, then finally straighten both legs and settle into pose. Heels will probably remain off floor. *Duration: 5 complete breaths, breathing slowly through the nose.*

(10) Plank to Chaturanga (*Chaturanga Dandasana*) - from Downward Dog come to Plank (push-up position). Inhale and bring your body a couple of inches off the floor and exhale pressing back to Plank. Hands placed under the shoulders or slightly wider, legs and abdominal muscles flexed. *Do this slowly 5-10 times.*

(11) Downward Facing Dog - from Plank, exhale and press back to Downward Dog again, *staying for 3 complete breaths.*

(12) Standing Forward Fold (*Uttanasana*) - from Down Dog bend your knees and as you exhale hop or step each feet forward toward your hands. Straighten your legs, keep your feet hip width apart, bring your back up parallel with the floor, and then exhale folding the torso over the legs. Keep your legs flexed with your weight evenly balanced on your feet from side to side and heel to toe, spine lengthening toward the crown of your head. *Duration: 5 complete breaths.*

(13 & 14) Standing Half Forward Fold (*Ardha Uttanasana*) - from Standing Forward Fold on an inhale bring your back up parallel with the floor, first extending your arms out to the side, then lengthening your arms out in front of you. Arms, back of head, neck and spine all in parallel alignment to floor. Keep your weight firmly balanced on your feet and extend out through your fingertips. *Duration: 5 complete breaths.*

(15) Standing Forward Fold - from Half Forward Fold, on the fifth exhale fold forward again into the full Standing Forward Fold. Keep legs flexed, weight balanced on feet, spine lengthened, neck relaxed. *Duration: 5 complete breaths.*

NOTE: *Repeat 12-15 two more times.*

(16 & 17) Transition to Standing - from Standing Forward Fold inhale and come up to Half Forward Fold with arms extended out to the side parallel with floor. On next inhale continue raising the torso, keeping the legs flexed and spine lengthened, sweeping the arms up from the sides of the body until the palms of the hands meet over head. Look to your hands above your head, and as you exhale extend the arms out to the side and down, bringing your palms together and lifting them to your sternum (heart) in a prayer gesture. *Stay here for 5 complete breaths.*

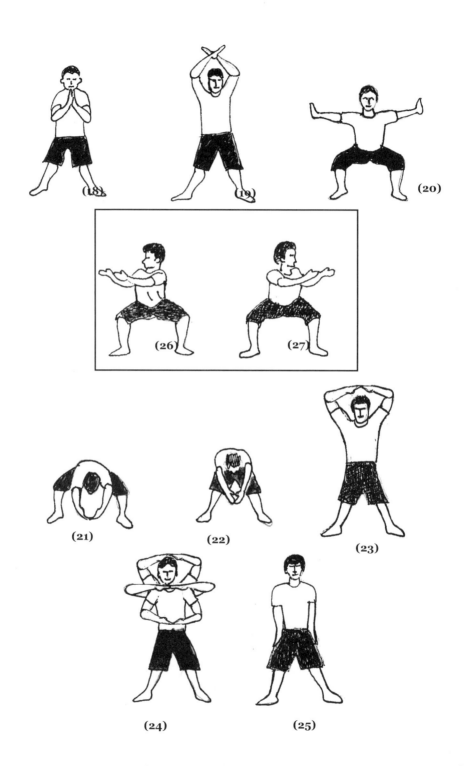

(18)

(19)

(20)

(26)

(27)

(21)

(22)

(23)

(24)

(25)

58

Purification (Taoist Flow)

NOTE: *The following sequence of poses 18-27 comprise a practice called Taoist Four Part Breathing .*

(18) Standing - begin with feet 3-4 feet apart, toes wider than heels, hands together at sternum in front of your heart.

(19 & 20) Arms Overhead to Squat - inhale and sweep your arms up, out to the side and over your head. Look up at your hands as your wrists cross over your head. Exhale and bend your knees, letting your legs and groin open out, working the energy meridian that runs along the inner legs. Extend the arms out to the side keeping your arms and hands flexed as you reach out through the palms. Keep your spine lengthened; chest open. Tailbone should be 4-6 inches higher than the knees. *Hold the squat at least 2 breaths before proceeding.*

(21, 22 & 23) Folding Forward to Standing – keeping your knees and legs bent, inhale as you fold your torso forward, bringing the hands together at the floor, with inner index fingers touching, tops of the hands facing outward. And continue the inhale as you slowly straighten your legs while drawing your straightened arms up from the floor out in front of you until your fingertips come together over your head. The entire motion as described is done on a single, full inhale.

(23 & 24) Drawing Energy to Core – with your arms raised over your head, fingertips touching, draw the energy down to the center of your body below the navel with your hands, keeping the elbows out to the side, palms facing the floor, fingertips touching, as you lower the arms and hands in a continuous, graceful motion.

(25) Standing - come to Standing arms alongside your body, feet 3-4 feet apart.

NOTE: *Repeat poses 18-25 six times, the forth time staying in the Squat (20) for 30-60 seconds, and the sixth time including poses 26 & 27.*

(26 & 27) Pulling the Bow - in one of the repetitions described above (18-20), while in the Squat (20), and before completing poses 21-25, bring the fingertips of your left hand to your right wrist and imitate drawing the string of a bow back along your inner arm to your heart. Repeat on the other arm, right fingertips to left wrist, drawing bow back to your heart. Then proceed to poses 21-25.

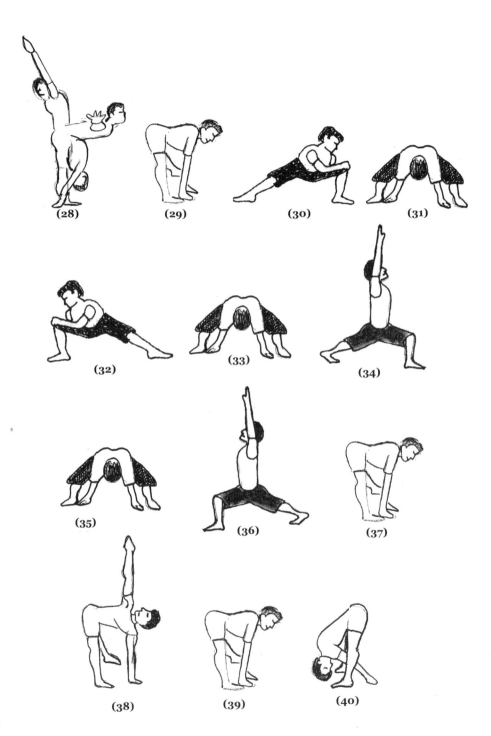

(28)　　　　(29)　　　　(30)　　　　(31)

(32)　　　　(33)　　　　(34)

(35)　　　　(36)　　　　(37)

(38)　　　　(39)　　　　(40)

60

Purification (Taoist Flow continued)

(28 & 29) Standing to Standing Spread Leg (*Padottanasana*) - after completing pose 25, bring your arms along side your body and straighten your feet where they are, keeping them 3-4 feet apart. Then upon inhaling, sweep your arms out to the side raising them to bring your hands together over your head. Look to your hands, and upon exhaling, fold forward keeping the spine lengthened while sweeping the arms downward, out to the side of your body. Bring the fingertips of your hands onto the floor under your shoulders.

(30, 31 & 32) Taoist Dips - while in the Standing Spread Leg **(29)**, take your feet at least 4 to 5 inches wider. Then inhale and as you exhale bend the left leg deeply as you move your torso over to the left. Drop the tailbone toward the floor and lengthen the right leg, keeping the right foot firmly planted on the mat. Then upon inhaling, transition to the other side, bending the right leg and keeping the left leg straight. Move with your breath, initiating movement on inhale, completing it on exhale as you bend the leg. Try to keep your tailbone low to the floor as you transition from one side to the other. *At least 5 repetitions each side.*

(33, 34, 35 & 36) Warrior (*Virabhadrasana I*) Lunges - as you transition from one side to the other in Taoist Dips, turn the foot of the bending leg toward the thin side of the mat, and keeping that leg bent, and the back leg straight, inhale and raise the arms over your head into Warrior I. As you exhale sweep the arms down and then across to the other side, and inhale and come up to Warrior I on that side. *At least 5 times both sides.*

(37 & 38, 39) Standing Spread Leg to Standing Spread Leg Twist - after completing Warrior Lunges, come back to Standing Spread Leg with your fingertips or palms touching the floor under your shoulders. Bring your right hand directly under your face, and while keeping your spine extended, inhale and twist the torso open to the left raising the left arm. Turn to look at your left hand. Exhale and bring left hand down under your face, then inhale and raise the right arm. Moving with your breath, alternate raising your arms. Engage your neck muscles so your head does not droop toward the floor. Keep your legs flexed. On your last repetition on each side stay in the pose with your arm raised for 30 seconds. Then come back to Standing Spread Leg.

(40) Standing Spread Leg Forward Fold - from Standing Spread Leg, walk your hands and arms under your legs keeping them shoulder width apart. Keep your arms straight, palms planted on the floor. Try not to round your back keeping the spine extended toward the crown of your head. Stay for 5 complete breaths before coming back to Standing Spread Leg **(39)**.

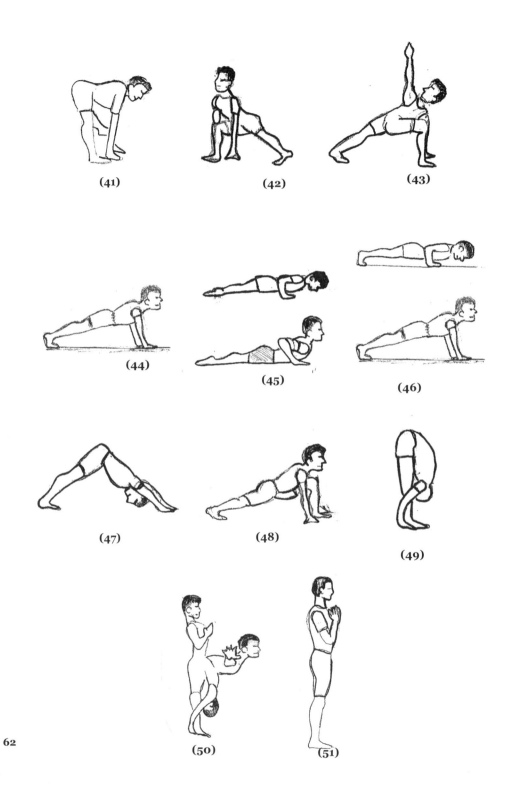

(41)   (42)   (43)

(44)   (45)   (46)

(47)   (48)   (49)

(50)   (51)

Purification (continued)

(41, 42 & 43) Low Lunge to Lunge Twist - from Standing Spread Leg start to move your upper body toward your right foot while pivoting that foot forward. Spin onto the ball of your left foot as you transition back to the Low Lunge. Then place the left hand under the left shoulder and twist your torso open to the right and extend your right arm and hand toward the ceiling. Keep the back leg straight, lifting up behind the knee. *Duration: 5 complete breaths.*

(44) Plank - from the Lunge Twist bring your right arm down and come back into the Low Lunge for a breath. Then step the right leg back and come into Plank (push-up position). *Stay in Plank for 2 complete breaths.*

(45) Cobra (Bhujangasana) - from Plank come down onto the floor resting your forehead on the mat. Bring your hands along side the pectoral muscles of your chest. Then flexing your gluteal (buttocks) muscles, keeping your legs and tops of feet pressed into the floor, on your next inhale lift your head and chest. The arms remain bent with elbows tucked in toward the ribs while drawing your shoulder blades down your back. Hands pressed lightly into the mat while lifting up from the sternum. *Duration: 5 complete breaths.*

(46 & 47) Plank to Downward Facing Dog - from Cobra come down onto the floor resting your forehead, staying for a breath, then curl your toes under and press up to Plank and back to Down Dog (see description pose 9). *Stay in Down Dog for 3 complete breaths, exhaling completely out your nose.*

(48) Low Lunge - from Down Dog, exhale and step the left foot forward into the Low Lunge. Prepare to repeat the Lunge Twist (43), this time raising the left arm, right hand on the mat under the right shoulder.

NOTE: *repeat poses 43-48 before doing 49, 50 & 51. When you repeat pose 48, the right foot steps forward into the Low Lunge from Down Dog.*

(49) Low Lunge to Standing Forward Fold - from the Low Lunge step the left foot next to the right and bring your back up parallel with the floor. Try to keep your fingertips in touch with the mat. Keep the legs flexed/straight; feet hip width apart. Inhale and as you exhale bend into the Standing Forward Fold. *Remain for 3 complete breaths.*

(50 & 51) Transition to Standing - from Standing Forward Fold, inhale and come up to standing with hands in front of heart (see description pose 16 & 17). *Remain here for 3 complete breaths.*

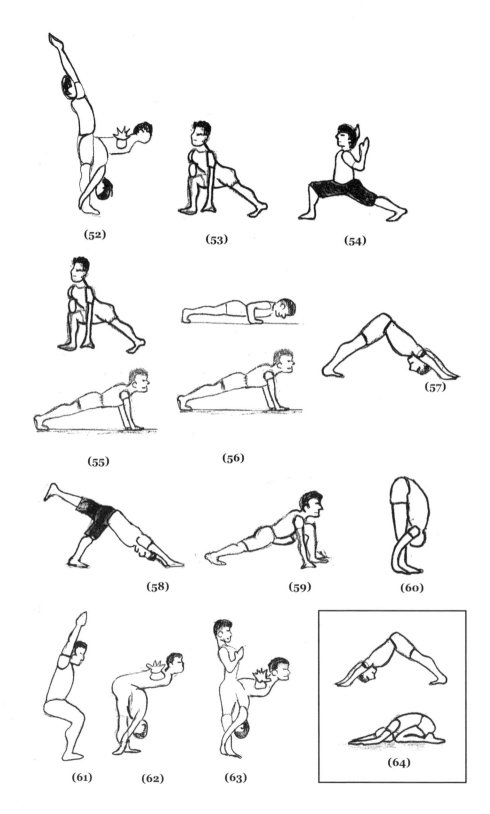

(52)   (53)   (54)

(55)   (56)   (57)

(58)   (59)   (60)

(61)   (62)   (63)   (64)

Purification (continued)

(52) Standing Forward Fold – from Standing with your hands together in front of your heart at your sternum (51), inhale and sweep your arms out to the side raising them so that your hands come together over your head. Look to your hands, and upon exhaling, fold forward keeping the spine lengthened while sweeping the arms downward along side your body and settling into the forward fold for *2 complete breaths.*

(53) Low Lunge - from Standing Forward Fold bring your back up parallel with the floor and as you fold your torso forward, step your left foot back into the Low Lunge.

(54) Standing Lunge ("Dragon Opens Its Wings") - from the Low Lunge, inhale and bring your head, chest and arms up with open hands. Arms are bent, elbows wide, chest open with shoulder blades drawn together. Keep the back leg straight lifting up behind the knee. Stay on the ball of the back foot and extend through the heel. *Stay 5 complete breaths.*

(55) Low Lunge to Plank - from "Dragon" exhale and place your fingertips down and come back into the Low Lunge for a breath. Then step the right leg back and come into Plank.

(56) Chaturanga to Upward Facing Dog (*Urdhvamukha Svanasana*) - from Plank come down a couple of inches off the floor to Chaturanga, then shift the chest and head forward while pressing upward to come into Upward Facing Dog. Lengthen the arms pressing the palms firmly into the floor under the shoulders. Lift from the crown of the head. Legs are flexed with knees off the floor, weight on the top of the feet, spine lengthening, look forward and slightly upward. *Stay 3-5 complete breaths.*

(57 & 58) Downward Facing Dog - from Upward Facing Dog shift onto the balls of your feet and exhale back to Downward Facing Dog for 2 breaths. Raise the left leg, flexing your left foot and lifting up from the heel. *Stay for 3 breaths.*

(59) Low Lunge - from Down Dog with your left leg raised, rise up onto the ball of your right foot and step the left foot forward coming into the Low Lunge.

(60) Standing Forward Fold - take a breath and from the Low Lunge step the right foot forward, hip width apart from the left foot, lift your back up parallel with the floor then fold forward over your legs to come into the Standing Forward Fold. Keep your weight balanced on your feet and your legs flexed.

(61) Powerful Squat (Utkatasana) - from the Standing Forward Fold, walk your feet together, bend your knees allowing them to come together. Your tailbone should be 4-6 inches higher than your knees. Inhale and sweep your arms up, shoulder width apart. Keep the tailbone tucked under. *Duration: 5 complete breaths.*

(62) Standing Forward Fold - from the Powerful Squat straighten your legs and bring your back parallel with the floor, arms out to the side to Standing Half Forward Fold. Then exhale folding forward into the Standing Forward Fold. *Duration: 3 complete breaths.*

(63) Transition to Standing - from Standing Forward Fold, inhale and come up to standing with hands in front of heart (see description pose16). *Remain here for 3 complete breaths.*

NOTE: *repeat poses 52 - 62. When repeating poses 53, 54 & 55 - the left foot is forward; right leg is back. Pose 58, right leg is raised in Down Dog. Pose 59, right foot is forward; left leg is back in Low Lunge. When you complete this second set of poses 52-62, rather than ending in pose 63, end in pose 64.*

(64) Downward Facing Dog to Child's Pose - from Standing Forward Fold (62) step the right leg back to the Low Lunge, then the left leg back into Downward Facing Dog. *Stay in Down Dog for 3 breaths, then come into Child's Pose for 10 complete breaths.*

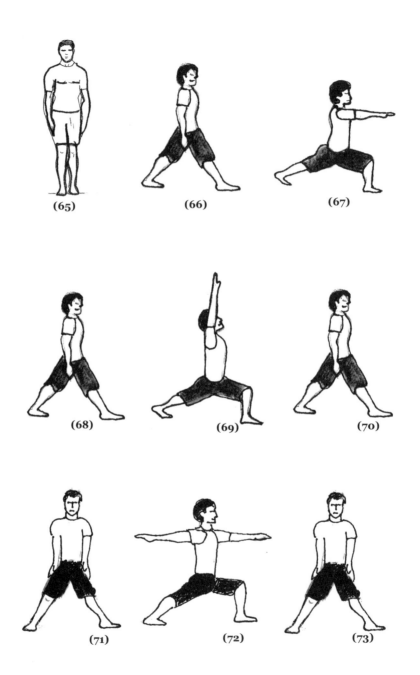

(65)   (66)   (67)

(68)   (69)   (70)

(71)   (72)   (73)

Resiliency (Warrior Standing Sequence)

(65) Mountain (*Tadasana*) - keeping your legs flexed, weight balanced on your feet, hip width apart, spine lengthened, shoulder blades slightly together and arms dangling along your side, close your eyes. Staying grounded through the soles of your feet, focus all of your awareness on the sensation of your breath moving in and out of the nose *Duration: 5 complete breaths.*

NOTE: *poses 66-70 are done as a continuous set.*

(66, 67 & 68) Warrior I Prep - from Mountain Pose step the right foot back 3-4 feet, keeping it angled forward. Try to maintain heel-to-heel alignment of the feet, from front to back. Hips should be squared, facing forward. Inhale and bend the left leg as close to 90° as possible while raising the arms chest high in front of you. Exhale and straighten the left leg while bringing your arms alongside your body. Repeat 4 times moving with the breath as described. *The fourth time hold pose 67 for 5 breaths before exhaling while bringing your arms alongside your body.*

(69 & 70) Warrior I (*Virabhadrasana I*) - from pose **68** (see description above), when next inhaling, bend the left leg and raise your arms overhead keeping the right leg straight and right foot firmly planted on the mat. Exhale and straighten the left leg while bringing your arms alongside your body (pose **70**). *Repeat 4 times, moving with the breath as described.* The fourth time hold pose **69** (Warrior I) for 5 breaths before exhaling while bringing your arms alongside your body.

NOTE: *Repeat poses 66-70 as described but with left foot back and right foot forward.*

(71, 72 & 73) Warrior II (*Virabhadrasana II*) - from pose 70 turn your right foot to the side, and open your hips in the same direction. Feet should be 4-5 ft. apart. Your front heel should be aligned with the middle of the arch of the back foot, the back foot angled slightly forward. Inhale and bring your arms up parallel with the floor as you bend the left leg as close to a 90° angle as possible. Your left knee should be directly over your left ankle. Keep the back leg straight lengthening it and pressing the back foot firmly into the mat. Look to the tips of your left fingers. Keep your torso vertically aligned over your hips. Exhale and straighten the left leg, bringing your arms alongside your body resting hands on thighs. *Repeat 4 times, moving with the breath as described.* The fourth time stay in pose 72 (Warrior II) for 5 full breaths before exhaling while bringing your arms alongside your body.

NOTE: *Repeat poses 71-73 as described but with left leg back and right leg forward, Look to right fingertips in pose 72.*

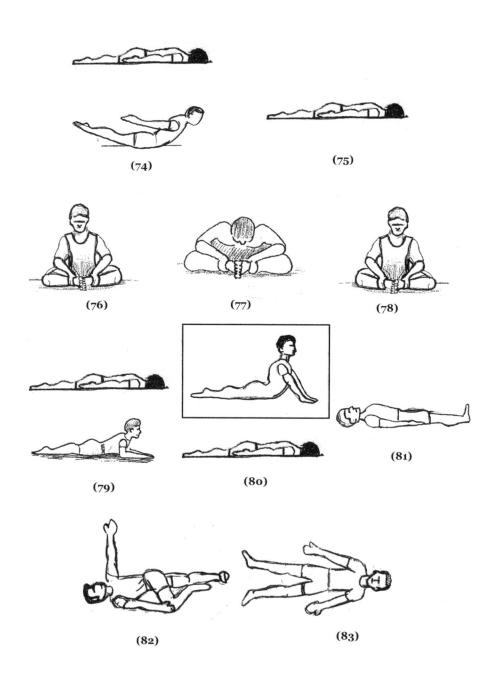

(74)

(75)

(76)

(77)

(78)

(79)

(80)

(81)

(82)

(83)

Closing & Integration

(74) Resting to Locust (*Salabhasana*) - after completing the Standing Sequence come lying down on your stomach on the mat, turning your head to the side. Take a couple of breaths, then on your next inhale lift your head and chest, lift your legs and extend your arms behind you. Keep your knees lifted, legs and feet close together and draw your shoulder blades together. Keep lifting up from the sternum. Duration: 5 complete breaths. *Do this 4-6 times, resting for 5 complete breaths in between going into the pose.* Alternate sides that you turn your head (left/right) when you come down to rest.

(75) Resting - come back to resting position with your head turned to the side.

(76) Cobbler (*Baddhakonasana*) - come to a seated position with the soles of your feet together, knees out to the side. Keep your back straight, spine lengthened. Stay for 3 complete breaths.

(77) Butterfly - while in Cobbler, move your feet forward 3-4º, about a foot in front of your knees, keeping the soles together. Inhale fully and as you exhale fold the torso forward over your legs, forehead dropping toward your feet. You can round your back. Let your chin rest on your collarbone. Keep your arms, shoulders and neck completely relaxed. Let the body surrender into the pose continuing to let go of any holding and tension. As you exhale in the pose draw your lower belly in toward your spine and keep the belly drawn in. Practice Mindful Awareness, let go of thinking and stay connected to your body and breath. *Remain in the pose a minimum of 3 minutes. With practice increase the time to 5 minutes.*

(78) Cobbler - from Butterfly slowly come up to Cobbler. You can stretch your legs out in front of you and lean back with your weight on your hands placed on the floor behind your shoulders. *Rest for a few breaths.*

(79) Sphinx – start by lying down on your stomach, head turned to the side. Stay for 3 complete breaths, then rise up onto your elbows and forearms. Elbows placed directly under the shoulders, arms resting on the floor shoulder width apart, legs and buttocks relaxed. Put a little pressure into your forearms and elbows so the chest does not sag toward the floor. Keep the belly soft. Practice Mindful Awareness, let go of thinking and stay connected to your body and breath. *Remain in the pose a minimum of 3 minutes.* With practice, increase the time to 5 minutes or move into Seal (pose 80) for the final 2 minutes.

(80) OPTIONAL: Seal - after being in Sphinx for 3 minutes, press your palms into the floor and straighten your arms. Keep the legs and buttocks relaxed. Be careful not to force yourself to stay in the pose if it feels like too much pressure on the lower back. Remain in Seal for 2 minutes before coming back down to Sphinx first before lying down and turning your head to the other side.

(81 & 82) Resting to Full Body Twist - from lying on your stomach roll over onto your back resting for 5 complete breaths. Then bend your left leg and with your hands on your left knee, bring it toward your chest. Step the left foot over to the outside of the right knee or thigh. Reach your left arm out to the left side along the floor, back of left shoulder in contact with the floor. Holding your left knee with your right hand, inhale and as you exhale, gently pull the left knee over to the right, bent left leg crossing over the straight right leg. Keep the back of your shoulders against the floor. *Remain for 1 minute.* Then come to lying on your back and repeat the pose as described with your right leg (crossing it over to the left, right arm reaching out to the right side).

(83) Corpse (*Savasana*) - after completing the Full Body Twist remain on your back. Separate your feet shoulder width apart and let the legs and feet roll open. Bring your hands about a foot away from the side of your body, palms open toward the ceiling. Walk your shoulders down away from your ears. Pick your head up, lengthen your neck and settle the head again. Let your body settle into a deep state of relaxation. Allow any pressure or tension from the scalp, forehead, temples, jaw to release to the floor where the back of your head rests. Let your body be completely held by the floor. Let your awareness remain with your breathing. *Stay for at least 5 minutes.* This is a good time to practice Deep Relaxation Breathing. End *Savasana* completely relaxed breathing naturally.

Warrior Practice

Centering & Opening

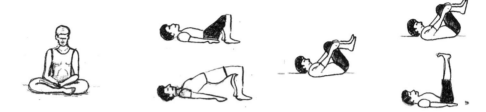

Opening (continued)

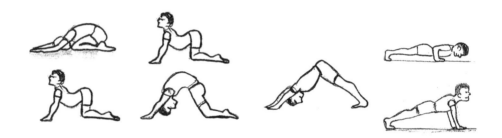

Purification (Taoist Flow)

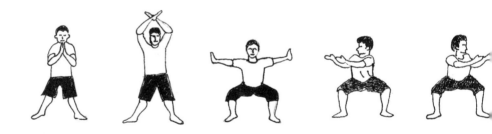

Purification (Taoist Flow continued)

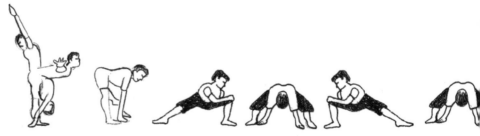

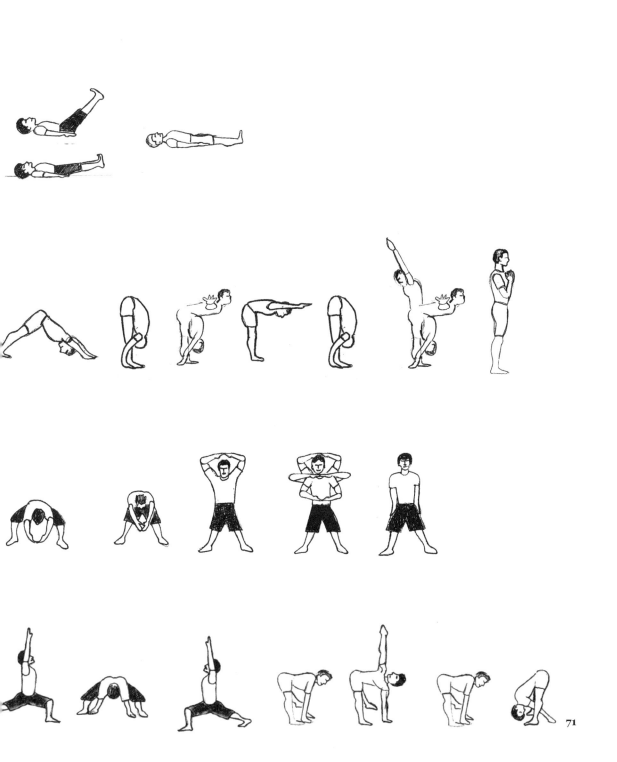

Warrior Practice

Purification (continued)

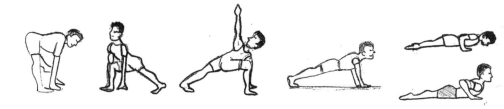

Purification (continued)

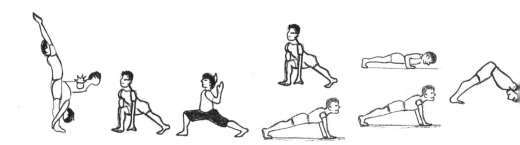

Resiliency (Warrior Standing Sequence)

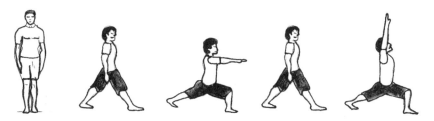

Centering & Integration

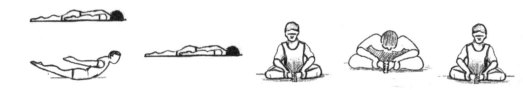

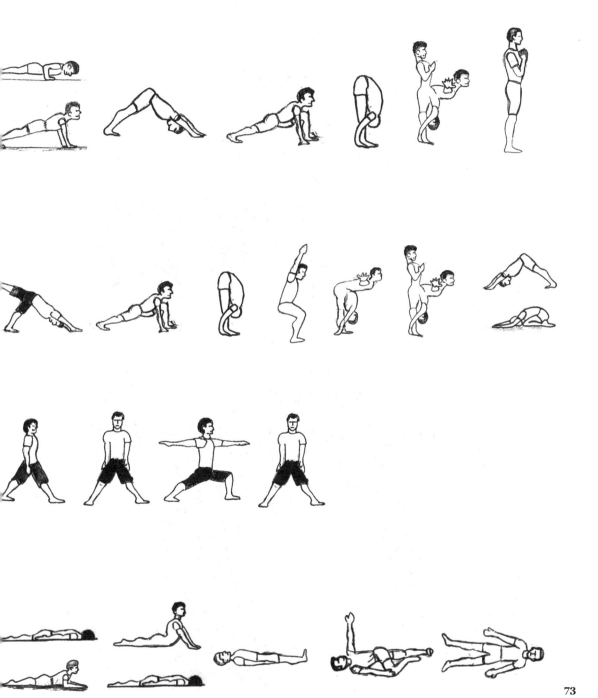

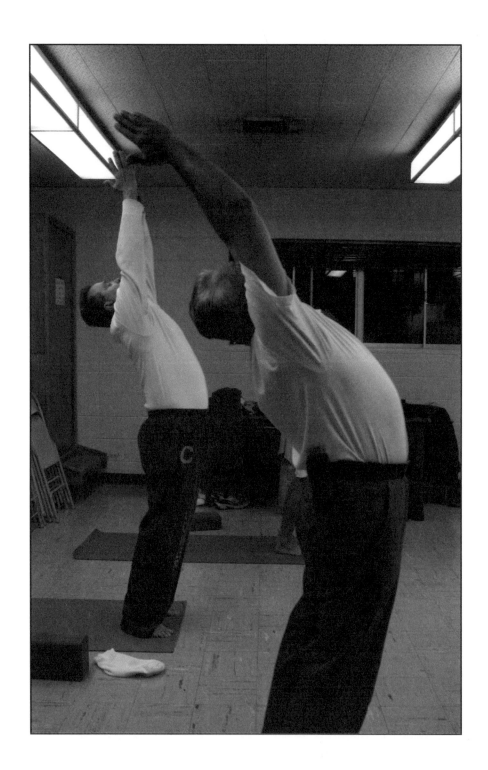

Quotes from Prisoners

I would like to thank you for your book. I have been practicing yoga for a year now and I am a firm believer that calming the mind is the single most important thing I have come to learn in prison. R.L., FCI Williamsburg, South Carolina

"Yoga A Path for Healing and Recovery" has changed my life completely. I put it aside at first because I was intimidated by it. But I read the book and started the process and have a beginning sense of real peace and clarity. Thank you from the bottom of my charkas. A.A., Stringfellow Unit, Rosharon, Texas

I just wanted you to know that your book did arrive to me, and I love it. I am handicapped (hands & legs) and there's not much to do here to maintain my health. Your book has already helped me reduce some of the pains, sleep easier and feel more alive with energy. A.H., Utah State Prison

I am on a path of spiritual freedom and release from the prison of self. I would like to request a copy of your book. My sincerest appreciation. B.D., Pennsylvania State Prison for Women

Some of us see that we need to take our rehabilitation into our own hands if we're going to make it. I'm glad folks like you are giving us some practical tools to work with. I look forward to receiving your book and putting it to use right away. W.T., Mule Creek State Prison, Ione, California

You recently sent me your book and it is a lifesaver. The years I have spent trying to find peace and relaxation that I have found practicing the exercises in your book. It's a miracle! K.M., CSP Solano, Solano, California

I wanted to thank you for the book. It is exactly what I was looking for to introduce me to yoga. I am anxious to share it with my family. M.K., Arkansas Dept. of Corrections, Malvern, Arkansas

I borrowed your book from my friend for a day. There was more power in two pages than I've experienced in ages. I'm very impressed and want yoga to become a part of my daily routine. Please send me a book at your earliest convenience. M.W., Ohio Reformatory for Women, Marysville, Ohio

The Fundamentals of *Pranayama*

Prana is the life force that permeates both the individual as well as the universe at all levels, and *ayama* is the storing and distribution of that energy. It is at once physical, sexual, mental, intellectual, spiritual, and cosmic. *Ayama* has three aspects or movements: vertical extension, horizontal extension, and cyclical extension. By practicing *pranayama*, we learn to move energy vertically, horizontally, and cyclically to the frontiers of the body.

The ancient yogis advocated the practice of *pranayama* to unite the breath with the mind, and therefore with *prana* or life force. *Pranayama* is not deep breathing. Deep breathing tenses the facial muscles, makes skull and scalp rigid, tightens the chest, and applies external force to the intake or release of breath. This creates hardness in the fibers of the lungs and chest, and prevents the percolation of breath through the body. In *pranayama*, the cells of the brain and the facial muscles remain soft and receptive, and the breath is drawn in or released gently. During inhalation, there should be no sudden movements. One becomes aware of the gradual expansion of the respiratory organs, and feels the breath reaching the most remote parts of the lungs in order to receive and absorb the *prana*. In exhalation, the release of breath is gradual, and gives the air cells sufficient time to reabsorb the residual *prana* to the maximum possible extent. This allows for the full utilization of energy, therefore building emotional stability and calming the mind.

The practice of *asanas* removes obstructions that block the flow of *prana*. During *pranayama*, one should be totally absorbed in refining the inhalation, exhalation, and in the naturalness of retention. One should not disturb or jerk the vital organs and nerves, or stress the brain cells. The brain is the instrument that observes the smooth flow of inhalation and exhalation. During breath cycles be mindful of the momentary pauses between the inhale and exhale, and the exhale and inhale, and a smooth flow will set in.

Learning about the Breath

Lengthening and holding your exhalation after the air is expelled relaxes you, while lengthening and holding in your inhalation energizes you. If you are feeling particularly stressed you are better off using a balanced breathing pattern. As you inhale let the belly, chest and ribcage expand without lifting your shoulders. Use the following as a guide.

Inhalation	Hold	Exhalation	Hold	Effect
4 counts*	1	8	1	Relaxing
8	1	8	1	Balanced
8	1	4	1	Energizing

*count = 1 second

Expanding Awareness of the Breath

EXERCISE (10-15 minutes)
Sitting on the floor with legs crossed or upright in a chair, back supported and feet flat on the floor, allow your eyes to close. Feel the weight of your body seated here in the chair. Notice that you are breathing. Breathing in and out of the nose, feel the natural rhythm of your breath as you inhale and exhale.

Then bring your awareness to your lower belly below your navel, and feel the belly as it expands on the inhale and contracts on the exhale (for at least 5 breath cycles of inhale/exhale).

Then bring your awareness to your diaphragm/solar plexus in between your ribcage, and feel the diaphragm expanding on the inhale and contracting on the exhale (for at least 5 breath cycles).

Then bring your awareness to your chest and ribcage and feel how the chest and ribcage expand on your inhale and contract on your exhale (for at least 5 breath cycles).

Now bring your awareness back to the natural movement of your breath as you inhale and exhale. Notice the overall expansion and contraction of the torso as you breath. Take several breaths doing this. Let your eyes open on a final exhale to complete the exercise.

Yogic Breathing - *Ujjayi Pranayama*

Ujjayi pranayama is one of the most commonly practiced yogic breathing techniques and represents a foundation for proper breathing while performing *asanas*. Unsteady breathing leads to an unsteady mind, therefore *Ujjayi pranayama* is practiced to calm the mind and body while harmonizing the rhythm of breathing.

Ujjayi pranayama serves three main purposes:
1) It helps to slow the breath down.
2) It focuses awareness on the breath and prevents the mind from wandering.
3) It adjusts the evenness and regulates the smooth flow of breath by continually drawing attention to the sound of the breath.

PRACTICE
Either lying down with your head supported by a pillow, or seated cross legged on a blanket or mat with your hips slightly elevated, begin by simply observing the natural flow of breathing through your nose for a minute or two.

Ujjayi breathing is introduced, first by extending the breath on the exhalation and then reversing that pattern, lengthening the inhalation while exhaling normally. To practice you can use an 8 to 4 count, first on exhalation to inhalation; then on inhalation to exhalation. Do not hold the breath in between inhales and exhales/exhales and inhales. In the final phase of the practice, you want to breath to an even count on both inhale and exhale (8 to 8). Keep the belly relaxed. As you inhale, allow the ribs and the chest to fully expand without raising the shoulders. When exhaling, let the exhale be complete following it with your awareness to its completion.

Then begin to inhale through your nose and exhale slowly through a wide-open mouth, directing the out-going flow of breath slowly across the back of your throat with a drawn-out "*hhhhha*" sound throughout the complete exhalation. Repeat several times, then close your mouth. Now, as you both inhale and exhale through your nose, direct the breath again slowly across the back of your throat, trying to make an "*hhhhha*" sound. Ideally, this will create, and you should hear, a soft hissing sound. Imagine that you are mimicking the sound of waves as they approach and retreat from shore.

Start with a 5 minute practice, gradually increasing to 10 minutes. When finished return to normal breathing for a minute or two, then lie down in *Shavasana* (Corpse Pose) for a few minutes. *Ujjayi pranayama* should also be used while practicing *asanas* to maintain a balanced mind and body, particularly during challenging moments.

Be careful not to use too much force. A sound that is too loud indicates too much internal conflict. Use the muscles of the throat lightly so that the energy within remains calm and pressure does not build around the temples.

Deep Relaxation Breathing - *Viloma Pranayama*

This is a slightly more advanced *pranayama* practice. It is recommended that you master the previous practices of Expanding Awareness of the Breath and *Ujjayi Pranayama* before engaging in *Viloma Pranayama*.

There are two types of *Viloma Pranayama,* also called Stop-Action Breathing. One focuses on the inhalation; the other on the exhalation. The following exercise with emphasis on exhalation is intended for calming the mind and body, releasing tension or anger, and experiencing a state of deep relaxation.

EXCERCISE (10-15 minutes)
Sitting on the floor with legs crossed or upright in a chair, back supported and feet flat on the floor, allow your eyes to close. You can also practice lying down if desired. This is a great pranayama practice before going to sleep, or when you awake in the middle of the night fighting demons in the mind.

Feel the sensations in your body, noticing where you are holding tension. Scan the body with your mind to discover exactly where you are tense. Then gradually bring your awareness/attention to your breath, breathing in and out of the nose. If you are stressed or agitated, you will notice a tendency of staying stuck in your mind. If your mind wanders or you become lost in thoughts, with kindness bring your awareness back to your breath, feeling the breath as it moves in and out of the body.

As you breathe, start to focus on your exhale, gradually letting all the air out of your lungs as you exhale completely. Continue to exhale completely, and make sure your exhale is twice as long, if not longer, than your inhale. Do this for 6-8 breathing cycles,

Then on your next breath, after exhaling completely, hold the breath to the count of 3 before inhaling. Keep repeating, hesitating before inhaling. While practicing be sure not to stress the body or tense the muscles of the stomach, diaphragm or chest. Let the breath flow smoothly. Do this for at least 10 breathing cycles. Then completely relax for a few minutes, allowing yourself to breathe naturally, aware of the rhythm of your breath.

Repeat the exercise if desired. Once you become familiar with it, you can practice this exercise whenever you feel tense or agitated. Remember to focus on exhaling completely. This triggers the parasympathetic nervous system, your relaxation response.

Breathing to Relieve Stress

EXERCISE (10-15 minutes)

Sitting in a cross-legged seated position or upright in a chair, back supported and feet flat on the floor, allow your eyes to close. If you wish, you can also do this exercise lying down on your back.

Feel the weight of your body seated or lying where you are. Breathing in and out of the nose, place your right hand on your belly below the navel with your left palm covering it. Tighten the belly then release it three times, taking a couple of breaths in between doing so. Then let the belly relax becoming soft and feel it rising and falling under your hands as you breath. Be aware that the lower belly about 2 inches below your navel represents the center of your body. Make sure that you exhale slowly and completely before inhaling. Do this for 10 breath cycles.

Then allow your eyes to open, and taking some full breaths in through your nose and out of your mouth, make an audible sigh upon exhaling (*ahhh*). Do this 8-10 times. Do not lift your shoulders as you inhale. Notice any area (throat, chest, diaphragm, belly) where you may be holding, gripping or where there is heaviness, and release it as you exhale.

Be sure to exhale completely as you sigh *ahhh*.

After you have completed this, close your eyes, return to your normal breathing, hands in your lap and just scan the internal energy of your body remaining aware of the natural movement of your breath. Do this for 1 minute before opening your eyes and completing the exercise.

You can repeat the exercise if desired.

Alternate Nostril Breathing - *Nadi Sodhana Pranayama*

Nadi Sodhana pranayama literally means "channel cleansing or purifying" breath. It is a more advanced *pranayama* practice that involves breathing alternately through each nostril. It is excellent for balancing right/left hemispheres of the brain, improving respiratory function and the level of oxygen in the blood, thus reducing stress, anxiety, depression and other mood disorders. It .can be a very useful breathing practice prior to moving into meditation.

PRACTICE
Seated in a cross-legged position or upright in a chair, keep your back straight and chin parallel to the floor. Using your right hand, fold the first two fingers of the hand into your palm. You will use your right thumb to close your right nostril and the inside of your right ring finger to close your left nostril. You want to close the nostrils at the top of the fleshy part where they meet the bone.

Bring your right hand to your face with the first two fingers bent in front of your nose, positioning your right thumb on the right side of your nose and the inside of the right ring finger along with the little finger on the left side of your nose. Close your eyes and exhale completely out your nose. Then gently close your left nostril with your right ring finger and inhale in through your right nostril. Then close the right nostril with the right thumb and breathe out your left nostril. Then breathe in through the left, close off that nostril with the right ring finger and breathe out through the right. That completes a "round." Begin practicing with a few rounds, then work up to a set of 12 rounds, which will likely take 2-3 minutes. After completing a set of 12 rounds, let yourself breathe naturally observing any mind/body sensations or changes that have occurred.

You want to feel comfortable with the pace, not too fast or too slow. Try to get a steady and equal rhythm going for both inhale and exhale, 4 to 5 counts each in duration. Each round ends breathing out the right nostril. If you become light-headed, slow your breathing down.

Once you have become accustomed to this practice, you can increase the number of sets (12 rounds) to two or three, allowing yourself to breathe naturally for at least a minute in between sets experiencing the mind/body effects of the practice.

Shining Forehead Breathing – *Kapala Bhati Pranayama*

This is an advanced *pranayama* practice that should be practiced with care and understanding. Do not perform *Kapala Bhati* until after you have mastered *Ujayii* and *Nadi Sodhana pranayama* practices.

Kapala Bhati Pranayama involves breathing in and out of the nose with emphasis on a forceful exhale while drawing in the stomach. The practice exercises internal organs, particularly the lungs, intestines, pancreas, liver and kidneys. It also strengthens the digestive and respiratory system, tones stomach muscles and stimulates the nervous system, increasing energy to the face particularly around the eyes and forehead. This is a good breathing practice for reducing stress, anxiety, depression and other mood disorders because of its oxygenating and increased energy effects. It .can also serve as a good *pranayama* practice prior to moving into meditation.

PRACTICE
Seated in a cross-legged position or upright in a chair, allow your eyes to close. Keep your back straight and chin parallel to the floor. Inhale allowing stomach to relax then exhale out the nose forcefully and completely while quickly drawing in your stomach (abdominal) muscles. It is somewhat like mimicking getting the breath slightly knocked out of you. Your inhale should be automatic requiring little effort. Your exhale should be strong, and will create a vacuum in the lungs that reflexively causes a short inhale. Try to complete 20-30 breath cycles (inhale/exhale) per minute.

Beginners can start by practicing in three, 1 minute rounds with 30 seconds of natural breathing in between. Over time and regular practice, build to 5 minutes of straight practice. Only after you have mastered 5 minutes of straight *Kapala Bhati Pranayama,* you can consider adding another 5 minute round, making sure to breathe naturally in seated meditation or light asana practice for 3-5 minutes in between the 5 minute rounds.

Caution: *Kapala Bhati Pranayama* should not to be attempted by pregnant women or anyone up to six months after surgery. Those with heart conditions or high blood pressure should practice gently. If you become light-headed, slow your breathing down and/or use fewer breaths for a lesser period of time.

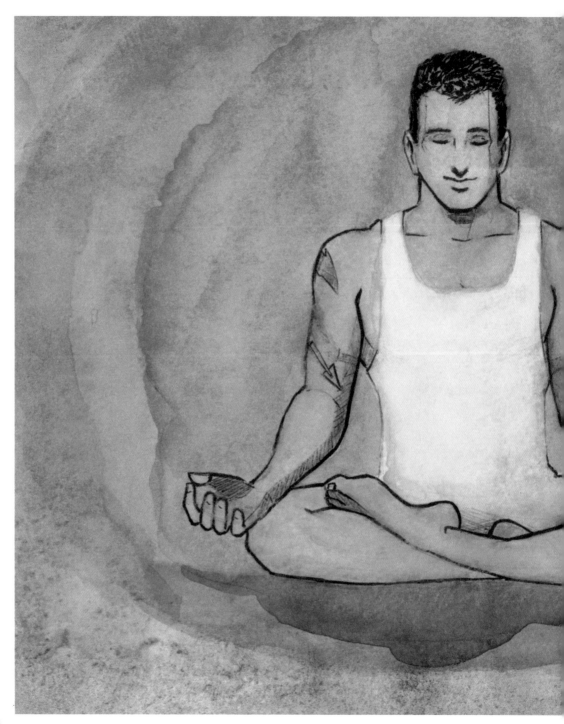

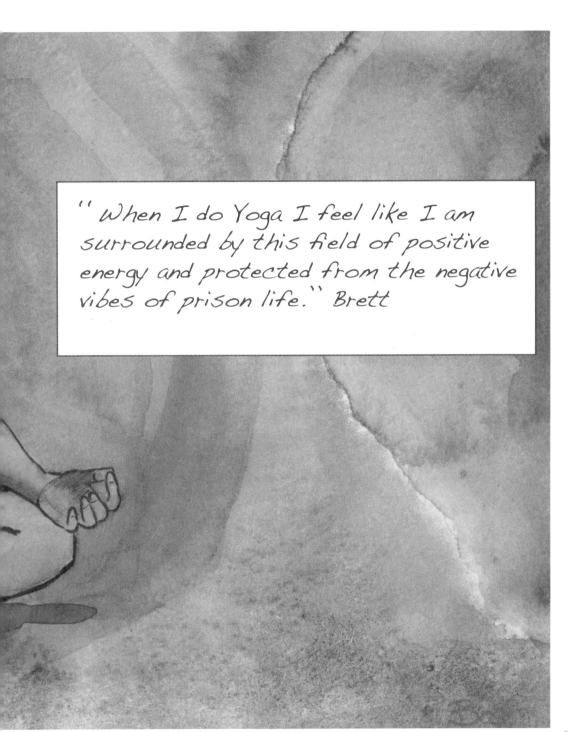

" When I do Yoga I feel like I am surrounded by this field of positive energy and protected from the negative vibes of prison life." Brett

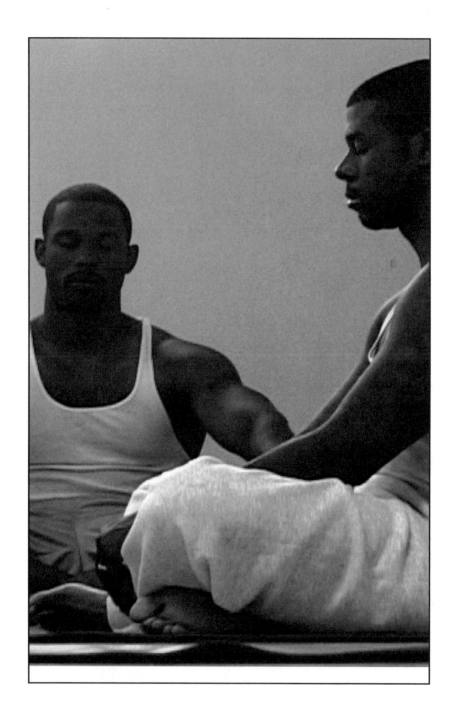

What Keeps Us from Experiencing Peace?

Peace begins with oneself. If one does not possess the ability and skills to remain clear and calm in the midst of life's challenges and stresses, then how can one effectively work in transforming conflict and violence into cooperation and peace?

A false sense of self is created by over identifying with the mind as who we are rather than with our true Being. Enslavement to incessant thinking brings about comparing, criticizing, disappointment, unhappiness, fear and suffering as a way of life. The mind habitually thinks that - one day when this or that happens - I will be happy, fulfilled and at peace. To be at peace requires us to break from this uniquely human pattern and condition by developing practices to stay connected with or conscious of our true nature. Yoga, meditation and Centering Prayer are among these practices. Art, music and other forms of creative expression can also foster a connectedness with Being.

Being is a state of oneness, a sense of recognition of who we truly are from deep within ourselves. Our Being is the knower behind the thinker; our innermost indestructible essence. The body, rather than the mind, can serve as a dependable point of access to Being. By disengaging from thoughts, observing our breathing, and connecting with deeper energetic sensations in our body, we can witness ourselves and the present moment as they truly are, free from the mind's interpretations.

Our Being is divine. The recognition of this as our true nature is our greatest attribute as peacemakers. The key to being at peace is to offer no resistance to what is. This does not mean not taking action. It means developing inner freedom by not reacting to external conditions. The compulsion to react comes from the mind's desire to control the outcome of situations.

When tension or negativity arise, pay very close attention to what is occurring in both your mind and body. See if you can stay out of your mind and experience the feelings associated with the situation in your body. Simply observe the feelings without becoming judgmental or attached to them. The mind wants to hold onto negativity thinking it can achieve a desirable outcome by doing so. But this is impossible since nothing positive can come from holding onto negative thoughts. This is why forgiveness is so powerful. Let the negative thoughts pass through you, becoming like light so there is no place for them to stick. Then, when you are firmly grounded in your Being, observing the present moment as it truly is, the steps and actions you need to take in the situation will become quite clear without the need for reactivity.

Daily Meditation Practice

Mindful Awareness or Mindfulness Meditation (20-30 minutes)

A daily meditation practice can help you to remain centered, connected to your authentic self, and allows for inner wisdom to arise.

First, choose a suitable space for your regular meditation. It can be wherever you can sit easily with minimum disturbance. Arrange what is around you so that you are reminded of your meditative purpose. You may want to make a place for favorite spiritual books, photos or cards.

Then select a regular time to practice that suits your schedule and temperament. If you are a morning person, sit before breakfast. If evenings fit your temperament or schedule better, try that first. Begin with sitting 10-20 minutes. Later you can sit longer or more often. Daily meditation can become like bathing, a regular cleaning and calming for your mind and heart.

Sit in a posture that reflects dignity without being rigid. Allow your spine to lengthen, shoulders relaxed, palms of hands resting on your thighs, or placed in your lap with the top of the right hand resting in the open upturned palm of your left hand, allowing your thumbs to touch gently. Let the tip of your tongue rest on the upper ridge of your mouth, behind your teeth. Let go of any worries, concerns, habitual thoughts. Feel your body seated where you are. Feel its weight. Find any tension in your body – face, neck, shoulders, belly – and let it go.

Then tune into the natural movement of your breath. Feel the breath as it moves in and out of the body, and feel the sensations in the body that accompany the breath. The rise and fall of the belly, the chest, the expansion of the ribcage, the sensation of the air as it moves through your nostrils. Let the breath be natural. Feel the sensations of the breath, relaxing into the breath, noticing how the soft sensations of breathing come and go with each inhale and exhale. Take a few full breaths sensing where you feel the breath most easily.

You will notice that after a few breaths your mind will begin to wander. When you notice this, no matter how long or short you drifted off on thoughts, simply bring your awareness back to the next breath. If you wish to, you can mindfully acknowledge where your attention had been by softly saying a word, such as "thinking," "remembering," "hearing," etc. Gently and directly return to feel the next breath. One word of acknowledgement and return to the breath is best. As you sit, let the breath change its rhythm naturally. Calm yourself by relaxing into the breath. When you become distracted by thoughts, gently bring yourself back to your breath, a thousand times if necessary. Be patient and kind with yourself. Over the weeks and months of this practice you will learn how to calm and center yourself using the breath. You will experience many cycles in the process, difficult days and more easy ones. Stay with it. As you do, deeply listening and feeling, you will be able to disengage from constant thinking and connect deeply with your body and spirit.

This meditation is an excellent foundation for working with the other meditations in this booklet.

From *A Path with Heart* by Jack Kornfield. Copyright ©1993 by Jack Kornfield. Used by permission of Bantam Books, a division of Random House, Inc.

Centering Prayer

The purpose of Contemplative Prayer is to open the mind, heart and whole being to God, beyond thoughts, words and emotions. By quieting our minds, stilling the body and engaging our will, we can open to an awareness of the Divine Presence within us entering into a state of consciousness in which we find our true self, thus finding God. Proponents of Contemplative Prayer teach that all human beings have a divine center and that all, not just born again believers, can discover their intrinsic goodness through the practice.

Contemplative Prayer is drawn from the early Christian prayer practices of the 4th Century, notably from the Fathers and Mothers of the Desert, from the Lectio Divina tradition (praying the scriptures), from works like The Cloud of Unknowing, and from the writings of St. John of the Cross and St. Teresa of Avila.

Centering Prayer is a practice designed to facilitate the development of Contemplative Prayer. Centering Prayer was introduced in the 1970's as an attempt to present the teachings of earlier times in an updated form by three Trappist monks: William Meninger, Basil Pennington and Abbot Thomas Keating at St. Joseph's Abbey in Spencer, Massachusetts. The purpose of Centering Prayer is to clear the mind of rational thought in order to focus on the indwelling presence of God. Centering Prayer places a strong emphasis on interior silence.

Guidelines for Practicing Centering Prayer (20-30 minutes)
1) Choose a sacred word that symbolizes your intention to consent to God's loving presence and action within you. Make it any word with particular meaning for your connection with the Divine, such as "Lord," "God," "Savior," "Abba," "Jesus," "Shalom," "Spirit," "Love," "Trust", etc.).

2) Sitting comfortably with your eyes closed, spend a minute or two to relax, allowing yourself to settle, dropping inwardly, and focusing on your breathing while letting go of thinking. Bring your awareness to your heart center at the sternum, feeling into your heart with your breath.

3) Introduce your sacred word and be gently present with your sincere intention to be in the Lord's presence and open to His divine action within you.

4) Whenever you become engaged in thoughts, emotions, bodily sensations, perceptions, images, associations, or any distractions from the practice – return, ever so gently, to your sacred word to anchor your intention to stay connected to God's presence.

5) At the end of the prayer period, remain with your eyes closed for a couple of minutes.You may wish to slowly recite the Lord's Prayer.

The minimum time for Centering Prayer is 20 minutes. Two periods a day are recommended: one first thing in the morning, and another in the afternoon or early evening, whichever best meets your schedule. With practice you may wish to extend the time to 30 minutes or longer.

During the Centering Prayer period ordinary wanderings of the imagination as well as thoughts and feelings may arise. You may experience psychological insights that arise from unloading the unconscious. Do not be discouraged. This is normal. When you notice you have gotten caught up in the current of thoughts, feelings, reflections, etc. – return to your original intention: Communion with God. Avoid analyzing your experience or aiming at a specific goal. Simply remain still resting in the awareness of your sacred word and rooted in your intention to connect with God.

Walking Meditation

Walking meditation is a simple and universal practice for developing calm, connectedness and awareness. It can be practiced regularly, on its own, or before or after sitting meditation.

The art of walking meditation is to learn to be aware as you walk, to use the natural movement of walking to cultivate mindful awareness.

Select a place where you can walk comfortably back and forth, indoors or out, ideally ten to thirty paces in length. This can become an excellent meditation practice for walking on the yard if you can train yourself to let go of distractions and stay within yourself. You can also use this practice in your cell. Even though it is a small space with few steps from one wall to the other, you can walk very slowly, and deliberately using the practice to center yourself and practice being present in the moment.

PRACTICE (20-30 minutes)

Begin by standing with you feet firmly planted. Let your hands rest easily wherever they are comfortable. Close your eyes for a moment, center yourself and feel your body in touch with the earth. Feel the pressure on the bottoms of your feet and the other natural sensations of standing. Then open your eyes and let yourself be fully present and alert.

Begin to walk slowly with a sense of ease and dignity. Pay attention to your body. With each step feel the sensations of lifting your foot and leg off the ground. Be aware as you place each foot on the earth. Relax and let your walking be easy and natural. Feel each step mindfully as you walk, particularly the soles of the feet as they contact the ground or floor. Pay attention to your breathing. You may wish to time your steps to your inhale and exhale.

If you are walking a straight path, when you reach the end of it, pause for a moment centering yourself. Carefully turn around and pause again so that you can be aware of your first step as you walk back.

If you are walking around the yard, simply stay focused on the bodily sensations of walking, the feeling of your feet contacting the ground and your breath. You can experiment with whatever pace keeps you most present.

Continue to walk back and forth for 10 to 20 minutes, or longer. As with the breath and sitting, your mind will wander many times. When you notice that you can acknowledge it softly by saying to yourself: "wandering," "thinking," "hearing," "planning," etc. Then return with awareness to the next step. Whether you drift off for a second or a few minutes, simply acknowledge that you have and come back to a full awareness of your next step.

After some practice with walking meditation you will learn to use it to calm and collect yourself, and live more fully in your body. You can extend your practice in an informal way as you walk to various places throughout your day. You will learn to enjoy walking as a simple way to be truly present, bringing your body, heart and mind together as you move through life.

From *A Path with Heart* by Jack Kornfield. Copyright ©1993 by Jack Kornfield. Used by permission of Bantam Books, a division of Random House, Inc.

Meditation Reflecting on Difficulty

PRACTICE (15 minutes)
Sit quietly, feeling the rhythm of your natural breathing, letting yourself become calm and receptive. Then think of a difficulty you are experiencing in your life. As you sense this difficulty, notice how it affects your body, heart and mind. Feeling it carefully, begin to ask a few questions, listening inwardly for answers.

How have I treated this difficulty so far?
How have I suffered by my own response and reaction to it?
What is this problem asking me to let go of?
What suffering is unavoidable, and which is my measure to accept?
What great lesson might this be able to teach me?
What is the gold, the value hidden in this situation?

In using this reflection to consider your difficulties, the openings and understandings may come slowly. Be patient and kind with yourself. As with all meditations, it can be helpful to repeat this meditation many times, listening each time for deeper understanding and answers from your body, heart and spirit.

From *A Path with Heart* by Jack Kornfield. Copyright ©1993 by Jack Kornfield. Used by permission of Bantam Books, a division of Random House, Inc.

Meditation on Stopping the War Within

You can engage in this practice for releasing the mental and emotional battles you have been waging inside of yourself.

PRACTICE (15-20 minutes)
Sit comfortably for a few minutes, letting your body be at rest, your breathing easy and natural. Bring your attention into the present and notice sensations in your body. In particular notice any tension, pain or sensations you may have been struggling with or fighting. Do not try to change them, simply notice them with interest and kind attention.

For each area of struggle in your life you discover, focus on relaxing your body and softening your heart. Open to whatever your experience is without fighting. Just breathe naturally and let it be.

Then after a few minutes, shift your attention to your heart and mind. Notice what emotions and thoughts are present. In particular notice any feelings or thoughts you are avoiding, fighting or denying. Notice them with interest and kind attention. Let your heart be soft opening to whatever you are experiencing without fighting. Let go of the battle; let it be.

Continue to sit quietly. Then bring your attention to all the battles that still exist in your life. Sense them inside you. If you have an ongoing battle with your body, be aware of that. If you have been fighting inner wars with your feelings, been in conflict with your own loneliness, fear, confusion, grief, anger, despair or addiction, sense the upset that you have been carrying. Notice the struggles in your thoughts as well. Be aware of how you have been waging inner battles. Be aware of all that you have fought and been fighting within yourself, and how long you've been carrying on the conflict.

Gently and with openness, allow these experiences to be present, noticing them with kind attention. In each area of struggle let your body, heart and mind be soft. Open to whatever you are experiencing without fighting. Let it be present just a it is. Let go of the battle, the constant struggling. Breathe quietly and let yourself be at rest. Invite your mind, heart and body to be at peace.

Loving Kindness Meditation

The following meditation is a 2,500-year old practice that uses repeated phrases, images and feelings to generate loving kindness toward oneself and others. It's best to begin by repeating it over and over for 15-20 minutes, once or twice daily, in a quiet place. At first it may feel mechanical or even bring up opposite feelings such as irritation and anger. If this happens it is especially important to be accepting and kind toward yourself, allowing whatever arises to be received with openness. Try doing this for several weeks, even months. With patience and practice it will calm you and keep you connected to your heart.

PART 1
May I be filled with loving kindness.
May I be healthy in mind and body. (or May I be healthy.)
May I be safe from internal and external danger. (or May I be peaceful and at ease.)
May I be truly happy and free.

PART 2
May you be filled with loving kindness.
May you be healthy in mind and body. (or May you be well.)
May you be safe from internal and external danger (or May you be peaceful and at ease.)
May you be truly happy and free.

TO BEGIN:
Sit in a seated position, on the floor with your legs crossed, or in a chair. Let your spine be straight, chest open, arms relaxed. Hands can be placed top of right hand in open left palm, or rest palms down on your thighs.

Connect with your body, feeling the physical sensations in the body. Then bring your awareness to your heart center at the sternum, feeling into your heart with your breath. Imagine that you are breathing in and out of your heart.

You, of all beings, are most deserving of your love. And, you cannot truly love someone else unless you love yourself. So, staying focused on your breath and heart center begin the practice (above) with yourself, repeating the words silently several times. Take your time. Stay focused on the breath and sensations at your heart. Let the feelings arise with the words. Repeat the phrases over and over. You can adjust the words and images to best suit you and open your heart of kindness. Practice this meditation for 5-10 minutes repeatedly for a number of weeks until the sense of loving kindness for yourself grows.

When you feel ready, in the same meditation period you can expand the focus of your loving kindness to others. After yourself, choose someone in your life who has truly cared about or for you. Picture them and recite the phrases substituting "I" with "you" (see above), repeating the words over and over, feeling into the heart with your breath. Do this for at least 5 minutes. After this you can begin to include others such as family members, friends or other people.

After you have practiced Loving Kindness Meditation on yourself and others you care about, you can choose someone with whom you have a difficult relationship and use the practice with this person. Staying aware of the breath and sensations that arise in the heart. When thoughts arise, re-direct your awareness to your breath and heart center. Notice the feelings in the heart center as you do the practice for at least 5 minutes.

When you get accustomed to this meditation practice you can do it anywhere, while waiting in lines, while walking and throughout your day. As you silently practice, over time you will no doubt feel a wonderful connection with yourself and others through the power of loving kindness.

Meditation on Forgiveness

Forgiveness enables us to be released from the sorrows of the past and allows for an easing of the heart. It can arise spontaneously or it can be developed. Like the Loving Kindness Meditation, there is a way to cultivate forgiveness through an ancient and systemic practice. Forgiveness can be used as a way to soften the heart and release the barriers to loving kindness for oneself and others. Through repeated practice we can bring the spirit of forgiveness into our lives.

Before doing forgiveness meditation, you must be clear about what forgiveness means. Forgiveness does not in any way justify or condone harmful actions. While you forgive, you may also say, "Never again will I knowingly allow this to happen." Forgiveness does not mean you have to seek out or speak to those who caused you harm. Forgiveness is an act of the heart, a movement to let go of the pain, resentment and burden you have carried for so long. We have all been harmed, just as we have all harmed ourselves and others.

For most people forgiveness is a process. When you have been deeply wounded the work of forgiveness can take years. It can go through stages: grief, rage, sorrow, fear, confusion. And if forgiveness is for yourself, for your own guilt, for the harm you've done to yourself or another, the process is the same. In the end if you can let yourself feel the pain you carry, it can come as a relief and release from your heart. You can discover that forgiveness is fundamentally for your own sake, a way to carry the pain of the past no longer.

THE PRACTICE (20 minutes)
Sit quietly, feeling the rhythm of your natural breathing, letting yourself become calm and receptive. Breathing gently into the area of the heart, let yourself feel all the barriers and holding that you have carried because you have not forgiven yourself or others. Let yourself feel the pain of keeping your heart closed. Then after breathing softly into the heart for some time, begin asking and extending forgiveness, opening your heart using the following words. Let the words, images and feelings grow deeper as you repeat them.

(1) Forgiveness from others

There are many ways that I have hurt and harmed others, betrayed or abandoned them, caused them suffering, knowingly or unknowingly, out of my own pain, fear, anger and confusion.

Let yourself remember and visualize the ways you have hurt others. Feel your own sorrow and regret and sense that you can finally release the burden and ask for forgiveness. Picture the memory that still burdens your heart, one by one, and repeat:

98

I ask for your forgiveness, I ask for your forgiveness.

(2) Forgiveness for yourself

Feel your own precious body and life, staying connected to your heart, and say these words:

There are many ways that I have betrayed, harmed or abandoned myself through thought, word or deed, knowingly or unknowingly.

Let yourself see the ways you have hurt and harmed yourself. Picture them, remember them, visualize them. Feel the sorrow you have carried from all these actions, and sense that you can release these burdens, extending forgiveness one by one to yourself. Then say to yourself:

For each of the ways I have hurt myself, through action or inaction, out of my own pain, fear, anger and confusion, I now extend a heartfelt forgiveness to myself. I forgive myself.

(3) Forgiveness for those who have hurt or harmed you.

Let yourself picture the times you have been hurt by others. Remember them; visualize them; one by one. Feel the sorrow you have carried from the past and sense that you can release yourself from this burden by extending forgiveness if your heart is ready. Now say to yourself:

In the many ways others (you) have hurt or harmed me, out of fear, pain, confusion and anger, I see these now. To the extent that I am ready, I offer them (you) forgiveness. I have carried this pain in my heart too long. For this reason, to those (you) who have caused me harm, I offer you my forgiveness. I forgive you.

Let yourself work with these three directions for forgiveness until you feel a release in your heart. Be patient and kind to yourself. It can take some time. Perhaps for some great pains you may not feel a complete release You may feel only the burden, anger or anguish you have held. Touch this gently. Be forgiving of yourself in this as well. Forgiveness cannot be forced; it cannot be artificial. Simply continue to practice, and let the words and images work gradually in their own way. In time, you can make the forgiveness meditation part of your regular practice, letting go of the past and opening your heart to each moment with loving kindness.

From *A Path with Heart* by Jack Kornfield. Copyright 1993 by Jack Kornfield.
Used by permission of Bantam Books, a division of Random House, Inc.

Writing Exercises

I invite you to use these exercises to write about your understanding and practice of yoga and mindful awareness while using this manual as a guide. There are ten exercises here. Each is intended as a weekly topic of focus and concentration for a course of study. However feel free to take whatever amount of time to reflect on these topics and write about them.

In having this book and more importantly using it, you are connected to a large sangha (Sanskrit for "community") comprised of thousands of other people, those incarcerated as well as many people on the outside who are involved with the Prison Yoga Project. This sangha is devoted to each other's highest good through our daily practice and the understanding of the topics of these exercises.

Please use separate pieces of paper or a journal to complete these exercises. And if after you've completed the course you wish to share any of your reflections or benefits you've experienced from your practice, please send them to: Reflections, c/o Prison Yoga Project, P.O. Box 415, Bolinas, CA 94924.

EXERCISE – WEEK 1

What is the meaning of "yoga"? Did you experience the union of your mind, heart and body this week? What does raja yoga mean and what are its origins? What are the three main practices involved in raja yoga?

EXERCISE – WEEK 2

How do you practice of Mindful Awareness? Are you able to experience it while doing your yoga practice? In what other ways have you been practicing Mindful Awareness?

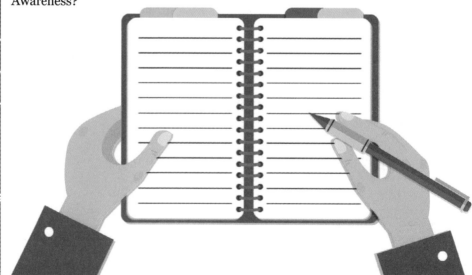

EXERCISE – WEEK 3

What are asanas? Which are your favorite ones? What is the meaning of prana? And what is pranayama? How do you use your breath to bring about relaxing effects? What is the sound you make to yourself when practicing Yogic Breathing? Are you able to practice Yogic Breathing while you do your asanas?

EXERCISE WEEK 4

What are the eight fundamental principles of raja yoga called? What is the principle for ethical behavior called? Please write about your understanding of the yamas and niyamas? Are they similar to other principles you know of?

EXERCISE - WEEK 5

What are chakras? What are nadis? How many chakras are there? Can you identify their location in your body?

EXERCISE – WEEK 6

With a focus on "A Deeper Understanding of Yoga," what is the traditional aim of the practice? Have you used the Meditation Practices (pgs. 87-98) in the manual? Which ones do you find most useful?

EXERCISE – WEEK 7

Do you see how "Self Image" is a mask, a false sense of self that hides you from your true identity? Can you see how your judgments keep you locked in a state of self-righteousness and unhappiness? Are you able to let go of thinking long enough to experience peace-of-mind?

EXERCISE – WEEK 8

What are the Two Levels of Perception discussed in the book? How often do you find yourself misinterpreting a situation or misperceiving a person? Do you understand the difficulty or suffering you cause yourself from this?

EXERCISE – WEEK 9

What is the Taoist word for vital life force energy? According to Taoist philosophy what are the two opposite yet interconnected forces of energy in the natural world? How do they balance each other? Are you able to bring them into your practice of yoga?

EXERCISE – WEEK 10

Now that you have been practicing regularly can you describe the overall benefits of yoga that you are experiencing? How do you use what you've learned from yoga in your daily life?

Recommended Books / Bibliography

Light On Yoga, B.K.S. Iyengar (Shocken Books)
The Spirit and Practice of Moving into Stillness, Erich Schiffmann (Pocket Books)
Insight Yoga, Sarah Powers (Shambhala Press)
Yin Yoga, A Quiet Practice, Paul Grilley (White Cloud Press)
Yoga: Conquering the Internal Nature, Swami Vivekananda (Vedanta Society)
Power Yoga, Beryl Bender Birch **(Simon & Shuster)**
The Heart of Yoga, T.K.V. Desikachar (Inner Traditions International)
Prayer of Heart and Body: Meditation and Yoga as a Christian Spiritual Practice, Thomas Ryan (Paulist Press)
Real Men Do Yoga, John Capouya (Health Communications)
Hatha Yoga Illustrated, Martin Kirk, Brooke Boon, and Daniel DiTuro (Human Kinetics)
Yoga for Body, Breath and Mind, A.G. Mohan (Rudra Press)
We're All Doing Time, Bo Lozoff (Human Kindness Foundation)
Houses of Healing: A Prisoner's Guide to Inner Power and Freedom, Robin Casarjian (Lionheart Foundation)
A Path with Heart, Jack Kornfield (Bantam Books)
A Gradual Awakening, Stephen Levine (Anchor Books)
The Power of Now, Eckhart Tolle (Namaste Publishing)
Tao Te Ching, Lao Tsu, translated by Gia-Fu Feng and Jane English (Vintage Books)

Namaste is a Sanskrit word with significant yogic meaning, commonly used in India as a greeting or acknowledgement to recognize the divine presence in each of us. The literal meaning of namaste is "I bow to you." In yoga it is most often spoken by teacher to students out of mutual respect and gratitude for one another at the beginning and/or end of a class. And students respond with the same greeting.

When speaking the word namaste, it is customary to bow the head with hands held together in a prayerful position at the heart. This allows for surrendering into the loving energy of the heart while acknowledging one's own soul and the soul of another as our true essence.

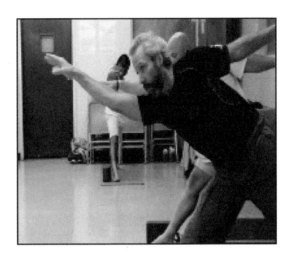

James Fox founded and directs the Prison Yoga Project. He is a certified yoga instructor and has studied and completed numerous trainings in various disciplines including Ashtanga, Iyengar, and Taoist Yoga, as well as Mindfulness Meditation over the past 23 years. Upon receiving his teaching credentials in 2000, in addition to offering classes to the public, he began his mission of exposing at-risk populations including the incarcerated to the psychological and physiological benefits of yoga.

James developed the Insight Prison Project's integrative health program at San Quentin State Prison that includes yoga and meditation, and has been its coordinator and principal teacher since its inception in September 2002. He has also taught yoga and Mindful Awareness practices to youth-at-risk in juvenile detention and residential treatment facilities. He is trained in the specific use of yoga for helping heal addictions. James is also involved in the Insight Prison Project's restorative justice (victim/offender education), emotional literacy and violence prevention work with prisoners.

Let us pray for healing, for strength,
for an end to pain and suffering,
and for goodness and peace in our lives.